MENOPAUSE
with Science and Soul

A GUIDEBOOK for NAVIGATING the JOURNEY

JUDITH L. BOICE, N.D., L.Ac.

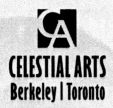

CELESTIAL ARTS
Berkeley | Toronto

Celestial Arts
an imprint of Ten Speed Press
PO Box 7123
Berkeley, California 94707
www.tenspeed.com

Distributed in Australia by Simon and Schuster Australia, in Canada by Ten Speed Press
Canada, in New Zealand by Southern Publishers Group, in South Africa by Real Books,
and in the United Kingdom and Europe by Publishers Group UK.

Cover design by Katy Brown
Text design by Lynn Bell

[Permissions acknowledgments:]

Library of Congress Cataloging-in-Publication Data
Menopause with science and soul : a guidebook for navigating the journey /
Judith I. Boice.
    p. cm.
  Includes bibliographical references and index.
  ISBN-13: 978-1-58761-291-6
  ISBN-10: 1-58761-291-7
  1. Menopause. 2. Middle-aged women—Health and hygiene.
3. Menopause—Miscellanea. I. Boice, Judith L. II. Title.

  RG186.M486 2007
  618.1'75—dc22

                          2006035662

Printed in the United States of America
First printing, 2007

1 2 3 4 5 6 7 8 9 10 — 11 10 09 08 07

CONTENTS

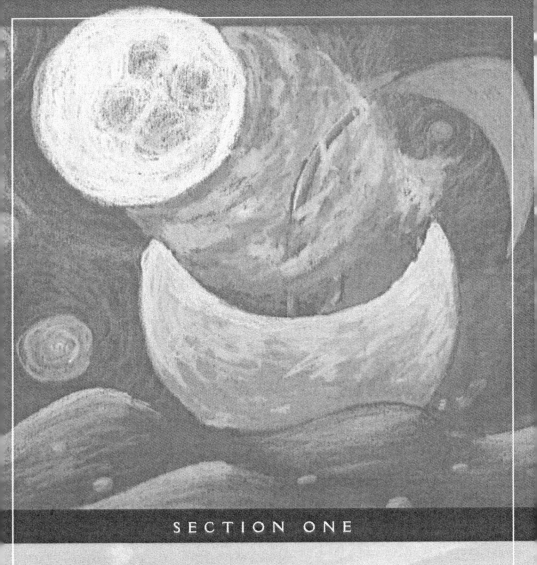

BEGINNING the JOURNEY

Prelude to Section One

"I want to take you on a journey," she whispers, motioning from the boat.

"But where are you taking me?" I ask hesitantly, eyeing this woman's dark, tattered clothes, her loosely braided gray hair, and the bone beads jangling on her chest.

"Why have you come to the river?" she asks.

I am annoyed that she answers my question with one of her own.

"I came for refreshment."

"You have come to be renewed," she corrects me. Her hand wraps around a rope on the bank of the river. Her grip is steady, patient. I realize I won't be able to decline the invitation. I could turn away from the river—temporarily. Eventually the river would come to reclaim everything: my home, my possessions, my life, my soul.

I step into the boat and sit on the aluminum seat of the bow. I want to face the river, to see what is ahead, but even more I am fascinated with this woman, so I sit facing her. I watch the way she deftly throws the rope into the boat. I observe how she digs an oar into the sand at the river's edge and pushes the boat from shore. Her muscular arms surprise me.

Every movement belies her intimate knowledge of this stretch of the river. I watch her eyebrows lift slightly in anticipation of a rapid; she instinctively digs an oar into the current to round a bend. Every muscle moves with precision, guided by familiarity and . . .

What? I pause, scrying her face, her thin-skinned, blue-veined hands. She moves with patience and weighted wisdom. Yes, wisdom I realize. She moves with the certainty of someone who has traveled this path many times. She reminds me of the elderly woman who has tended children all her life and can anticipate each developmental stage of an infant, a toddler, a preschooler. Her charges, though, are much older. This is the child's development in reverse. I am embarking on the journey of aging. The baby is preparing for life; I am preparing for death. The revelation startles me. The baby accrues life, gathering the bulk of flesh and experience around itself. I am dropping all that is extraneous. This is aging in reverse. I am entering the infancy of cronehood.

Suddenly, in her presence, I feel young and protected. My thigh muscles relax a bit against the seat. I can shift my gaze to the banks of the river and appreciate the scent of pine trees and patterns of river rock strewn in the currents. Yes, this will be a journey, I decide. Yes, this River Woman knows the currents. She will be my guide. My shoulders recede from my ears. Yes, I decide. I can trust her.

Poem by Clarissa Pinkola Estès

Dr. Clarissa Pinkola Estès is an author, poet, and psychoanalyst. Her books include Women Who Run with the Wolves *and* The Faithful Gardener.

The Red Room — The Hysterectomy

Gone is the tiny room they came to.
From far star roofs
they once jumped, giggling.
Tiny travelers with no baggage
came here,
hoping to find
all they needed.
And I brought some here safely.
Now, the waiting room is gone.
This station is closed.

But a thousand other rooms
that once seemed sealed with steel bands
I find now are only held shut with
cellophane.
I find that there are rooms between
rooms in me,
and they can open fully.

If, as in the days of my child-bearing years,
I let this ancient rope
with child attached grow in me, then when ready,
let it slip through and from me into life outside,

if I do not hold too tight, but rather loosen
all the bracelets of my body, letting these
new ideas come in their own time,
just let what I know have its ways
with me, as always before.

The red room is gone.
But the runway lights are still lit
fully blue
glowing
in this darkness
that grows revolution,
that welcomes visitors
blazing with life.

CHAPTER ONE

PREPARATION for the JOURNEY

THIS IS THE VERY BEGINNING OF THE JOURNEY, THE PREPARATION PHASE, when you haul out the suitcase or backpack and begin to sort through the items you plan to bring with you. The size of your luggage, however, prompts the discarding phase. "Will I *really* need sixteen pairs of underwear for a ten-day trip? How important is my yellow vinyl rain hat in Arizona? Will I need *1001 Car Games for Kids* with my sixteen-year-old son?"

You may begin to realize that this journey will require more releasing than accumulating. How much personal or cultural paraphernalia will you really need? Do your personal beliefs about this menopausal journey serve you? Have you even sorted through the legacy of stories, facts, opinions, and prejudices that have shaped your personal expectations about this life transition?

Years ago I was preparing to leave Scotland for India. At least a half dozen people in the community where I lived approached me to share *their* experiences of traveling in India. The majority spoke of stolen suitcases, swindled money, illness, filthy toilets, and assaulted women. By the time I arrived in India, I was so frightened I could not sleep. I rode twelve hours on the bus without getting out to urinate. (I wasn't ready to face the toilets yet.) I arrived at my destination exhausted and sick from the physical tension I carried in my body. I lived in southern India for almost five months. Only in the last month did I finally relax and enjoy my stay.

I know my friends were trying to help me with their cautionary tales. What I really needed, though, was inspiration along with the warnings. I certainly needed an antidote to my naïveté about traveling in third-world countries. What I did *not* need, however, was to have them squelch my joy and anticipation about traveling on a new continent, in a new world.

I hope to offer you the same blending of reality and possibility, risk and revelation in your own menopausal journey. None of us can know exactly what will befall us on the trek. We can, however, share our stories—the mishaps as well as the triumphs—and thereby garner wisdom and affirmation for our own personal journey.

MENOPAUSAL SYMPTOMS

Many women in this culture experience a host of symptoms (see list below) as they transition through menopause. For some, the passage is a horrific, nightmarish journey. For others, "the Change" sparks "menopausal zest," increased energy, and a newfound sense of freedom.

Just as each woman is individual in her experience of menopause, so is she unique in the support she will or will not need. About 15 to 20 percent of women in this culture breeze through menopause with no symptoms whatsoever. In many other cultures, the reverse is true: menopausal symptoms are rare. Two groups that have been studied precisely because women have so few menopausal symptoms are Japanese women in Asia and indigenous Mayan women in South America.[1] These are not the only cultures in which women experience few or no menopausal symptoms, but they are two that have been researched. Most Asian languages, for example, have no word for "hot flash" because hot flashes simply are not part of Asian women's experience.

Sally came to my office very distressed after seeing her HMO physician, an older Asian woman. According to Sally, the HMO doctor "... had no sympathy for what I'm going through *at all*." While Sally described her

---

Symptoms Associated with Menopause:

- Hot flashes
- Night sweats
- Dry skin and hair
- Thinning hair
- Vaginal dryness
- Vaginal atrophy (thinning of vaginal tissue)
- Memory lapses, especially short-term memory
- Insomnia
- Decreased sexual desire
- Indigestion
- Increased food allergies
- Increased inhalant allergies
- Depression
- Increased hair growth on face and body
- Panic attacks
- Migraine headaches
- Flatulence
- Osteoporosis
- Decreased thyroid function
- Sore heels
- Urinary tract infections
- Irritability, nervousness, anxiety
- Sore breasts

debilitating hot flashes and a host of other menopausal symptoms, the Asian doctor "looked at me as if I were from Mars."

"Your doctor probably didn't mean to be unkind," I said. "She just literally had no idea what you were talking about." As an Asian woman, the doctor had no cultural context to understand this patient's experience.

You are not required to have any of the long list of symptoms that can accompany menopause. You also are not "wrong" to have symptoms. Just keep in mind that symptoms are optional.

The good news is that you do have some influence over your menopausal experience. At least five factors play into whether or not you will have symptoms, and three of the five are in your control.

1. Genetics

Genes determine the *time* a woman will go into menopause, but they do not dictate the quality of the passage. Women enter menopause around the same time as their mother, maternal grandmother, and maternal great-grandmother. A mother's experience of menopause, however, does not necessarily determine her daughter's experience. Just because my mother had severe hot flashes, for example, does not automatically mean that I will have severe hot flashes, nor does a mother's lack of symptoms guarantee a smooth passage for her daughter.

Certain factors can speed the transition into menopause. A major physical or emotional trauma, for example, can catapult a woman into menopause. Chemotherapy and certain other drugs can stop ovarian function and push a woman into an early menopause. This "chemically induced" menopause can occur within months of beginning drug therapy. Surgery can also force an early menopause. After removing the ovaries (oophorectomy), menopause occurs quickly, within twenty-four hours. Other surgeries may catalyze the transition into menopause simply by increasing stress levels in the body. Removing the uterus (hysterectomy) may also hasten the shut down of the ovaries, as removal of the uterus can disrupt the blood supply to the ovaries.

2. Diet

Nutrition plays a major role in a woman's menopausal experience. Obviously the more unprocessed, fresh, whole foods a woman eats, and the more appropriate her diet is for her particular body, the more nourished she will be during her menopausal transition. Japanese and traditional Mayan women probably are not living on Big Macs and Hamburger Helper. Their diets include locally grown fresh foods, with a minimum of processed or "junk" foods. Chapter 7 discusses specific dietary recommendations for menopausal women.

In Japan, phytoestrogens play a major role in a woman's diet. In chapter 5, we will take a closer look at the impact of phytoestrogens on women's health. Phyto- means "plant," so phytoestrogens are plant molecules that *mimic* but do not exactly duplicate your body's estrogens. Phytoestrogens, in fact, are 400 to 1000 times weaker than the estrogens your body produces. Plant-based estrogens still have significant estrogenic activity, but they are much weaker than the estrogens you make. Although they cannot substitute for an estrogen prescription, phytoestrogens offer many benefits for menopausal women.

3. Exercise

In contrast to most North American women, Japanese and Mayan women probably do not have to join a gym to get their daily exercise. Instead, exercise comes as part of their daily lives. They walk to the store, work in the house and garden, and generally are much more physically active than most North American women.

Exercise can be a powerful ally during menopause. One study in this culture demonstrated that women who exercise aerobically at least 3.5 hours a week have about 75 percent fewer hot flashes.[2] Exercise supports your body in many other ways, too, by improving sleep, reducing stress and anxiety, and increasing bone mineral density.

Consider ways to incorporate exercise in your daily life. Usually the more effort required (e.g., putting on Lycra tights, driving to the gym, exercising, taking a shower), the less likely you will be to continue exercising on a regular basis. See chapter 8 for more specific information about exercise for menopausal women.

4. Xenoestrogen Exposure

Xeno means "foreign," so "xenoestrogens" are foreign substances that have estrogen-like activity in the body. Xenoestrogens do not exactly duplicate the estrogens you make, yet they affect estrogen-receptor sites. You can inhale, ingest, and/or absorb xenoestrogens through your skin. Examples of xenoestrogens include chloro- and fluorocarbons, insecticides, and pesticides. Off-gassing from plastics, such as those in new cars, carpets, draperies, and furniture, releases xenoestrogens that you absorb through your lungs. Heating plastics in microwave ovens causes the plastic to migrate into whatever it contacts, in this case the food or drink it holds. You can absorb chlorine through your steamed-open pores when showering in chlorinated water. Fluorescent lighting ballasts often contain PCBs, potent xenoestrogens, that can affect those exposed to artificial lighting.

In this culture, we tend to have lots of xenoestrogen exposures. "Better living through chemistry," the battle cry of the 1950s and '60s, has had a profound effect on our health. Researchers find traces of chemicals no longer sold in this country years after our last exposure, for example, DDT in our fat cells and in mothers' breast milk. Our body stores chloro- and fluorocarbons in fat cells and lymphatic tissue. Breasts and reproductive organs—both men's and women's—are mainly composed of fat and lymph tissue. The recent "epidemic" of breast and testicular cancers is hardly a mystery—our bodies concentrate fat-soluble carcinogens in these tissues.

Rather than pouring millions of dollars into cancer-treatment research, we could more effectively spend that money eliminating toxic pollutants, one of the chief causes of reproductive cancers. A cursory look at environmental conditions in the areas of highest cancer incidence provides major clues about the cause of cancer. The San Francisco Bay area, for example, has one of the highest breast cancer rates in the United States. Emissions from a rubber tire–burning plant drift into the Bay Area, effluents from silicon processing plants pollute the waters, and oil refineries line parts of the bay. Xenoestrogens literally bombard men and women in the San Francisco Bay area, a fact sadly reflected in the region's cancer statistics.

The pulp and paper industry uses dioxins, chlorine-containing compounds, to bleach paper products white. Tampons, for example, are bleached-white paper products laced with dioxins. We place them against the vaginal wall, one of the most absorptive tissue surfaces in the body. In 1994, the Environmental Protection Agency (EPA) cited dioxin TCDD (tetrachlorodibenzo-p-dioxin) as the most toxic substance known to humanity.[3] In addition to mimicking estrogen and modulating hormone levels in the body, dioxins also significantly reduce the immune response in the body, increase risk for breast cancer, and contribute to reduced sperm counts in men.

Xenoestrogen Sources

- Polychlorinated biphenyls (PCBs) are directly related to breast cancer. Trade names include Arochlor, Clophen, Fenclor, Inerteen, Kanechlor, and Phenoclor.
- Chlorinated water
- Fluorescent lighting (often contain PCBs)
- Dioxins
- Insecticides and pesticides, e.g., DDT and its breakdown product, DDE
- Off-gassing from plastics
- Heated plastics (e.g., in microwave ovens) containing food or beverages
- Bisphenol-A, the precursor of polycarbonate plastics, commonly found in lubricants, toiletries, detergents, and spermicides

Eliminating dioxins and other organochlorine chemicals could significantly reduce cancer rates. "Ten years after the Israeli government outlawed the use of three major organochlorine pesticides (lindane, benzene hexachloride, and DDT), breast cancer rates dropped by 30%. This decade of decreasing breast cancer rates was preceded by 25 years of steadily increasing breast cancer occurrences."[4]

Because of high xenoestrogen exposures, North American women tend to have relatively higher estrogen activity than Japanese and Mayan women. The prolonged elevation in estrogen activity increases the incidence of "estrogen dominance" symptoms, which we will discuss in more detail in chapter 4.

5. Personal and Cultural Attitudes about Aging

In Japanese, Mayan, and most indigenous cultures, both men and women gain social stature as they age. They are more respected, more honored, and more revered. Most women in this culture have the polar opposite experience: they feel they are losing something, diminishing both in social stature and respect. This culture tends to view elders as disposable goods unworthy of attention. We ignore the strengths—experience, wisdom, perspective—that elders bring. Most of us value physically measurable production, not such intangibles as insight and knowledge. This culture goes beyond admiring youth to wholesale worship of nubile forms. We expect people, particularly women, to look like twenty-two-year-olds all their lives. We do not attempt to halt the progression from childhood to adolescence, yet we have a cultural fear, reflected in current medical practice, of advancing into our elder years. I have never heard of physicians trying to halt a child's hormonal progression into puberty, yet those same practitioners chivalrously devote themselves to blocking a woman's transition through menopause. The medical community preys on cultural vanity and plies women with estrogen, promising wrinkle-free youthfulness for all takers.

The cultural disgust for elders may mask our fears: we tremble at the prospect of aging in our physical bodies. To a certain extent, this apprehension may be justified. Our culture is rife with ageism. Many women divulge their fears of growing older during office visits. During a recent phone consultation with a highly educated, upper-management executive, we discussed natural or "bio-identical" progesterone and other options for hormone replacement therapy (HRT). "I'm on this Premarin stuff," she explained, "and I'm going crazy, but I just *have* to keep taking it."

"If you are having so many side effects," I asked quietly, "why are you still taking the estrogen?"

"Because I can't afford to look old!" she blurted, tension rising in her voice. "I'll lose my job. I can't afford to lose this job. At my age, in this industry, I'll never find another one!"

My fury rose as I listened. My anger was not directed at this woman, but rather at a society that forces a woman to choose between physical health (she knows the dangers of hormone replacement therapy) and financial survival. Many menopausal women feel torn between sane health-care decisions and economic or social survival. Women fear losing partners, families, jobs, and/or economic security. I was angry at the internalized oppression that causes women to make choices that may damage their health, even kill them, in pursuit of a youthful appearance.

From studies in this culture, we know that the more relaxed and in control a woman feels, the fewer hot flash symptoms she will have.5, 6 A woman entering menopause in a culture that does not value elders is less likely to feel she is in control. In a culture that disregards elders, that treats them as nuisances to be tolerated, no wonder women have so many menopausal symptoms!

A network of family and friends can provide invaluable support for a menopausal woman. Women are different on the other side of menopause, just as girls are different moving from childhood into adolescence, and adolescence into adulthood. We change. Often menopausal women are more direct and outspoken. They say what they want to say and do what they want to do. A network of family and friends who welcome these changes is an invaluable asset for a menopausal woman.

Pawnee Chinn, a long-time friend, was well informed about menopause, so hot flashes and other physical changes did not surprise her, but "the freeing of thinking and feeling did. Emotionally I noticed I gradually felt different. I let go of worrying about the details of my life: looking a certain way, doing things a certain way, and even thinking a certain way. Menopause freed me up to be more of who I really am. I notice now when my husband and others are thinking and doing what they *think* is expected of them instead of what they want. I 'go along with' now *much* less than before. It doesn't go well with some people, but the beautiful thing is *I don't care.*"

In some cultures, this life transition is an important time for reflection and reevaluation. Women have raised families, developed careers, and accomplished many things by this time in their lives. Women's focus shifts from the immediate needs of family or coworkers to the larger community.

"How do I want to use my time? In what ways can I serve the larger society?" asks the woman approaching her elder years. Or, as my friend Julia Turner (see her reflections on page XXX) reminds me, after years of caring for others, the question is "What do I want to do for ME?"

Take time to acknowledge what you have accomplished, the journey that has brought you to this place. When you have a clear view of the path that led you here, consider how you would like to shape your future. What do you want to do with the rest of your life? What do you want your life to look like in twenty years? forty years? Often some of the richest, most satisfying, most rewarding years still lie ahead. Chart your course. Mark your goals. Envision the world you wish to live in. The journey will continue whether you choose to navigate or not. You have an opportunity to influence the direction of that path. See chapter 2 for guidance on creating your health goals and chapter 12 for more information about marking and celebrating this life passage.

Genetics, diet, exercise, xenoestrogens, and attitudes about aging all influence a woman's passage through menopause. Certainly these five are not the only important factors, but they are major influences on a woman's experience of menopause. The good news is that at least three of the factors are completely in your control: what you eat, whether or not you exercise, and your attitude (which affects the mental/emotional support network you develop).

You can minimize xenoestrogen exposures by eating organic foods and eliminating pesticides from your lawn and garden. Filtering water can reduce chlorine exposure. On a larger scale, you can reduce xenoestrogens by supporting responsible, environmentally sound industry in your local region. Healthy people live in a healthy environment, so everything you do to support the environment in turn supports your own health.

MENTORS ON THE JOURNEY

Shortly before my due date for completing this book, my root-cellar office flooded. The previous owner had dug the root cellar deep enough to stand in, poured a concrete floor, added carpet and drywall, and cut skylights into the ceiling. I use this special "hobbit hole" for writing. The root cellar is also cluttered with boxes and papers that have not been unpacked since the boys and I moved here over five years ago. I had been planning to tackle this mountain of unsorted papers after the manuscript was complete. Instead, heavy rains and a clogged drain forced me to haul the sodden mess out of the root cellar into my back hallway. That rainy Sunday afternoon, I spread soaked toddler photos of my sons all over the living-room floor. I sorted old letters, including the last letters my grandmother wrote before Alzheimer's spirited away her mind. I reread letters from college friends, filled with the intensity and passion so tangible during that transition into adulthood. Over the next week, I reconnected with the many roots that support the tree of my life.

A mentor pointed out the perfection of the "root cellar" reconnecting me with my biological and spiritual "roots." I realized the interviews collected for the book were in part a gathering of my own spiritual roots, drawing upon the women who have been friends, allies, mentors, and honored elders on my own journey.

These women's stories represent a broad range of menopausal experience, to illustrate that each woman's journey is unique, that there is no one "right" way to transition through menopause.

I am deeply moved by the wisdom these women have shared. Each is dedicated in her own way to serving others, and these interviews are examples of their generosity of spirit. I am deeply grateful for these gifts of wisdom. My own journey is much richer because of their sharing.

May their reflections—or the reflections of elders from your own line-age—illuminate your path and inspire you to draw upon them for more wisdom and guidance. Each interview includes contact information so that you can continue the conversation, if you so desire. May their words recon-nect you with your *own* wisdom, the ultimate source of renewal.

Gathering Support for the Journey Ahead

Before each session of writing this book, I would spend at least half an hour in meditation. One golden September afternoon, as I sat before the key-board, a woman entered my consciousness, much like a waking dream. She guided me to the river and a waiting boat. She is River Woman who intro-duces each section of this book.

River Woman quickly became a guide in many areas of my life. She appeared in meditations and dreams. I sense her even now as I write. I've come to know her as a guide and mentor during this season of my life. I realize now that focusing my attention on menopause, particularly the spiri-tual aspects of the journey, invoked her presence in my life.

River Woman also became a guide for the book, serving as navigator for the stages of the menopausal journey. She reinforced how each stage of the life journey "dies" into the next. If I move consciously through these transi-tions, the life I am leaving behind becomes fertile soil for the next phase of my life. I am learning to embrace that process of death and transformation instead of fearing the changes that menopause can bring. River Woman as well as many of the women interviewed in the book echo that understand-ing of "dying" into a new way of being, a new stage of the life cycle, rather than clinging to the old.

I invite you to make space within yourself for a guide, mentor, or teacher to become manifest in your life. That wise being may take many forms. You may have an experience similar to mine, with a guide who dwells in the nonphysical world. You may encounter a new friend or teacher, very much alive and well in physical form. An animal, plant, or color may ally itself with you. This being may first enter your dreams, your meditations, or your neighborhood diner. The possibilities are endless. The main point here is to open your heart and mind to wisdom and guidance.

I offer the following meditation as a beginning point in welcoming a mentor and guide into your life. If nothing "happens" in the meditation, please don't despair. Many inner experiences are like seeds planted in the soul, and have a way of growing—sometimes predictably and sometimes in any unruly tangle—into our outer, physical life. The wisdom moves into us with a pacing and presentation that is perfect for each of us individually. Make way for the muse to surprise you with her wit and wisdom.

I encourage you to begin a special journal to record your experiences during your menopausal journey. Over the years, I have developed several journals, one for my dreams, another for meditations, and a third for daily observations. You may choose to create separate journals or keep one notebook that combines all of your musings in one place. I think of my journal as a spiritual companion, a confidante on my journey. I am amazed when I look back, sometimes years later, at the wisdom and insight recorded in these journals. I wish I were as wise in my "waking" world as I am in my dream and meditation worlds!

Research on creativity confirms that recording observations, ideas, and inspirations spawns more creativity and inspiration. I'm reminded of the Native American teaching story about what we feed inside ourselves. If we feed fear, anger, and hopelessness, we foster a desolate soul. If we feed inspiration, wisdom, and insight, we nurture the creative, life-affirming aspects of our lives. Keeping a journal, or recording observations on a tape recorder, reinforces the wise, creative, vital aspects of our lives.

Any book—a spiral notebook or a hand-bound book—will do. Waiting to find or buy "the perfect journal" may guarantee that you never will begin. I encourage you to choose something simple and easy so that you can start right away.

MEDITATION

Note: you may choose to record this meditation on a cassette tape so that you can relax more fully during the meditation. The initial grounding meditation may be incorporated into any of the meditations presented in this book.

Set aside at least twenty minutes when you will be uninterrupted (no telephones, children, cats, or other disruptions). Place your journal next to you so that you can easily record your experiences when you emerge from meditation. Sit comfortably on a chair or cushion, with your spine straight.

Take a few deep breaths, close your eyes, and allow any surface tension in your body to melt away. Take a few moments to notice the flow of air moving in and out of your lungs, passing gently in and out of your nostrils. With each breath, allow your body and mind to relax more deeply.

Place your attention on your "root chakra," an energetic center that, for women, resides approximately between the ovaries. Some women sense this area at the base of the spine or in the vaginal region. Trust your body sense.

From the root chakra, send a chord or a root downward, through the floorboards beneath you, into the soil. Allow that root to grow downward through the thin layer of soil into the bedrock. Continue sending that root deeper into the earth, through the molten layer of rock, right to the very center of the earth. When you arrive at that center, allow the root to grow firmly around that central core.

Allow any tension, dis-ease, or fatigue to flow down this chord into the earth. This "negative" energy from your body is food for the earth. Like composted broccoli stems and coffee grounds, the earth will transform the "garbage" into nourishment and vitality.

Sense now that you are drawing nourishment up this root into your body. Just as a plant absorbs water and food from the soil, bring the earth's nourishment into your physical body. Allow that energy to fill the root chakra, and then spread outward to vitalize every cell of your body.

When you are filled with the earth's energy, sense yourself reaching upward from your crown chakra, at the top of the head. Grow upward into the stars. Bring that celestial energy into the top of your head. You may visualize or imagine golden light cascading downward, bathing every cell in your body. Allow the energy of the heavens to mingle with the energy of the earth.

See or imagine yourself walking through a forest. You can do this very easily. Notice the trees around you, the leaves beneath your feet. Move through the woods until you find a path winding among the trees. Follow this path into a meadow. Notice how you feel as you enter this sunny, warm, open space.

Take a few moments to explore the meadow, walking easily until you find a comfortable spot to sit down. Relax in this delightfully comfortable place in the meadow.

Remind yourself why you have come to the meadow. You are seeking a mentor, guide, and teacher for your menopausal journey. Ask from the deepest, wisest place inside for the perfect support during this phase of your life journey.

Relax and notice who or what enters the meadow. Allow any expectations of what you will discover to come into your mind . . .and then pass away like clouds drifting across a windy, spring sky. Be open to the unexpected.

Keep in mind you always have control of what you will accept or reject in this space. You are in control of this meadow space. If you are not comfortable with any person or being that enters the meadow, you are always free to ask them to leave.

Gift yourself with several minutes to relax in this meadow. You will easily recall all of the events that occur on this trip to the meadow.

When your experience is complete, open your eyes and record what you have experienced in the meadow. Keep your journal close by, as you may receive more inspiration and guidance in the days ahead.

Reflections by Carol Bridges

Carol Bridges has been leading women's empowerment groups since 1976 and currently teaches feng shui at her Nine Harmonies School. She is the author of The Medicine Woman Tarot, The Medicine Woman's Inner Guidebook, A Soul in Place, The Code of the Goddess, The Medicine Woman's Guide to Being in Business for Yourself, *and* Secrets Stored in Ecstasy. *Carol currently focuses on her art and creating sacred space in the environment.*

In my thirties, I attended a radical therapy conference where two menopausal wise women shared their idea that menopausal hot flashes were simply the sacred, spiritual kundalini energy rising. They explained that we get two spiritual boosts in our lives, one at adolescence and one at menopause. During these times of drastic self-image alteration, we get a gift of extra juice in order to create the life we want for the next phase of our time on earth.

I remembered this wisdom when my own "power surges" started happening. Although I had been consciously pursuing my spiritual path for many years, I appreciated that my body would no longer allow me to tolerate any conditions in my life that I really did not like. I think that if we have created a fairly satisfactory life, at least the angry flares and/or total depression that sometimes accompany menopause are greatly minimized.

One of the things I had to do all of a sudden (or so it seemed) was move to California. Even though I later returned to my present home in Indiana, the move put me in communion with a large social circle of women who shared my view of the world and who were themselves wildly creative. There I felt very much supported.

Fortunately I suffered no extreme physical or emotional side effects of menopause. I never use medical drugs or any other mood-altering substances except meditation, art, and fun. Through a process I call "shamanic journaling," I retold my life story to myself several times, just to make sure I was telling myself a version that would allow me to age gracefully. Creating collages of one's past history and changing a few details can be a very liberating experience—no use carrying around excess baggage of past events. Just dismantling the cultural stereotype of aging is challenge enough.

A lot of achievement occurred during my menopausal years, even a bit of fame and public appreciation for things I have done. My financial situation was better than ever. My partner (currently a twenty-two-year relationship) was totally at peace with my life stage even though he is nine years younger. My three sons were off living their own lives. I had been doing my heartfelt work in the world for most of my adult life. Sounds perfect, doesn't it?

I am deeply grateful for all of these blessings. But I don't want to imply that the shift from appearing youthful, especially in a culture focused on young sexuality, is in any way easy as we see our appearance changing. "Who is that in the mirror, anyway?" Just when everything is going right and we finally have become comfortable with ourselves, we begin to look "old." Another hurdle to overcome. What is natural to aging anyway?

The culture provides almost no images of beautiful elders living interesting lives. If there is anything I would have wished for, it would have been a culture that values all body types and ages and does not pretend that drugs and surgery are the answer. A well-known medical doctor said that before our generation all menopausal research was done on men and dogs! So we are the groundbreakers, doing our own research and expanding the limits. As I look at photos of my grandmothers in their late fifties, I see we are at least twenty years younger in looks, health, and attitude. Last year, at 63, I built my first room addition all by myself after never having done more than hang a picture! I know I do ten times the physical work that I ever did in my twenties, even though I had three children under three at that time. We are changing the aging picture!

My personal wisdom gleaned from my years of menopausal experience is that if we have done pretty much what we wanted to in our lives, we will just refine that path. If, however, there are areas where we were too timid, or the situation prevented us from expressing ourselves, or we gave too much in some area of responsibility, the menopausal energy will not let it rest.

The hot flash, angry outburst, or breakaway must happen or severe disease results. I am fortunate. My spirit was always strong enough to let go of unbeneficial situations after a good try at making things better.

How has my spiritual tradition helped me? My belief that the Holy One resides in my own heart has given me the ground of self-respect necessary to create a life that is deeply satisfying. I also learned in early childhood to be grateful for every little thing, for nothing is so small that God does not reside therein.

I see the elder years as a time of great freedom to deepen this relationship to the beauty, the God/Goddess-in-All-Things, around me. Menopause says, "If not now, when?" Do what you love. This really is it.

Carol can be reached at www.nineharmonies.com.

CHART YOUR COURSE: CREATING YOUR PERSONAL VISION of HEALTH

"WHEN YOU GO TO THE BUS STATION," EXPLAINS PHYLLIS RODIN, A ninety-two-year-old friend, "you've got to know where you're going before you can buy a ticket. The same thing is true in your life: you've got to know where you're going before you can buy a ticket. That's the ticket!"

Most office visits with a doctor begin with questions about where you are: "What is the problem? Where are you hurting? How long have you had this problem?" When new patients come into my office, I first ask where they want to go: "Do you want to be healthy?" Often patients give me a perplexed look.

"But I'm here for my digestion," exclaimed one woman.

"Yes, I understand that from your intake form. First, though, I'd like to know if you want to be healthy, and if so, what health looks like for you."

Over the years I have learned that some people want to be healthy, and others do not. Initially almost everyone says, "Of course I want to be healthy!" After realizing how much time and effort might be involved, however, many change their minds. Rather than judging someone's decision, I support a patient's freedom to make choices regarding her health, including the choice not to be healthy.

If the answer is "Yes," the next question is "What does health look like for *you?*" Each woman has her own individual vision of health. During our first office visit, part of my mission is to encourage a patient to paint her own individual picture of health.

One of the first secrets in journeying toward health is choosing to be healthy. Have you chosen to be healthy?

CHOOSING HEALTH

As you consider whether or not you want to be healthy, ask yourself, "*Why* do I want to be healthy?" Most people have never asked themselves this question. "Well, of course I'm supposed to want to be healthy," you may say to yourself. "Doesn't everyone want to be healthy?"

For most people, health is a necessary prerequisite to create what truly matters to them. Without health, they cannot bring those visions to fruition.

Motivation

Consider what is most important to you in your life. What matters to you? What do you want to create? For the moment, set aside thoughts about whether or not those creations are possible; instead, tell yourself the truth about what you really want in life.

Although many people desire health, each person has her own reason for wanting to be healthy. For Ann, choosing health may be a way of pleasing her spouse. Carolyn may choose health to avoid heart disease or cancer. Sarah Jane may desire health so that she can create what matters most to her. Paula may choose health to support her life vision of raising a family and pursuing a painting career.

Your motivation for choosing health impacts your ability to create health. Choosing health to serve your life vision fundamentally differs from avoiding illness, problem solving, or pleasing others.

Pitfalls on the Journey to Creating Health: Avoiding, Problem solving, and Placating

Consider again the original question: Have you made a choice to be healthy? Many women pursue all kinds of "health programs," dietary approaches, and exercise routines, yet they have never chosen to be healthy. These women may choose to participate in programs to *avoid* certain illnesses or to avoid losing their health. When they avoid something, however, what do they end up with? The *absence* of something. Remember that full, vibrant health is more than the absence of disease, more than the avoidance of future illness.

Problem Solving versus Creating

Creating something is radically different from problem solving. When you solve a problem, the difficulty "goes away." Instead of creating something new, you have eliminated something you do not want. You are left with nothing.

Most medical systems focus on eliminating problems: Slay the symptom. Avoid illness. Prevent disease. All of these approaches are problem-solving strategies. None of these methods focus on what you want to create; instead, they address what you want to avoid or eliminate. As you create health, you may very well employ medical services to fulfill your vision of health. The framework in which you apply those treatments, however, varies completely from the problem-solving approach.

Avoiding the Ravages of Disease

My friend Mary called shortly after her annual gynecological exam with the news that her physician had found a breast lump. She wanted me to verify her physician's explanation of the mammogram report.

"Here are the test results," she said, reading them over the phone. "Is my doctor telling me the truth, or is he trying to make me feel better so I don't worry?" Filled with medical jargon, the mammogram report basically stated that she probably had an aggressive, malignant tumor. The physician could not make a definitive diagnosis until after he had completed a biopsy of the tumor.

During the following month, Mary's life changed radically. Her tumor was malignant, and she had reams of decisions to make. In addition to having surgery to remove the breast lump, Mary changed her diet and began a natural supplement regimen. She decided to pursue chemotherapy treatments but refused radiation because of its poor track record in treating her particular type of cancer.

One Saturday afternoon Mary called in a panic, wanting to know if she could take more of the acidophilus supplement her doctor had recommended. She was struggling with candida overgrowth in her vagina and on her skin that caused tremendous itching. Chemotherapy wipes out all the flora in the digestive tract, providing the perfect environment for certain bacteria and fungi to flourish. I tried to refer her back to her own doctor, but she was insistent.

I explained that the doctor probably had recommended taking only a small amount of acidophilus rather than following the full program because she would wipe out the flora all over again with the next round of chemotherapy.

"Will taking more acidophilus hurt me?" asked Mary.

"No," I explained, "but you're wasting your money. Your doctor suggested you take a small amount because the next round of chemotherapy will destroy the microorganisms you are replacing now."

"I understand I'm probably wasting my money taking more of the acidophilus," said Mary, "but what can I do *now?*"

I empathized with Mary. "Chemotherapy is amazing stuff," I said. "It shuts down everything in the body. That's its nature. Chemotherapy stops all cell division, in the tumor and in the rest of the body."

"Well, I didn't really have any choice," she said, sighing.

"It's your body, isn't it?" I asked.

"Yes," she said, "but my family was totally freaked out when I told them I was thinking about not doing chemotherapy. They just wouldn't listen to me. I *had* to do this."

"Does your body belong to you or your family?" I asked again.

"It's more complicated than that," she replied.

Mary is right. We often face extremely complicated health-care decisions, particularly if we are struggling with a chronic or terminal disease. Many women who have been healthy all their lives face medical problems for the first time during perimenopause and menopause. Breast cancer, low thyroid function, weight gain, high blood pressure, heart disease, uterine fibroids, endometriosis, and a host of other conditions are more prevalent during this stage of the life cycle. Remember that no one is *required* to have any of these illnesses. In later chapters, as we discuss the effects of various hormones and how the levels change during perimenopause and menopause, you will understand why these diseases *can* affect more women.

Mary hoped to elude the cancer *and* avoid her family's distress about her health-care choices. Usually we are busy trying to avoid undesirable circumstances. Rather than moving toward a vision of health, we are running desperately from a feared condition.

"Solving the problem" of breast cancer (or any other condition) will not necessarily create health. Someone with breast cancer, however, could choose to create health. The fact that she has breast cancer becomes part of the evaluation of her current health status. Breast cancer becomes a feature in the landscape rather than the sole focus of her attention.

Some women with breast cancer can create their vision of health, while others cannot. Women with breast cancer or anyone else with a serious illness will have a greater chance of creating health if they desire health in order to fulfill other important life goals. Rather than solving the problem of cancer, their health-care choices support the creation of what truly matters to them.

Resolving a Problem Will Not Create Health

Ellen, another woman diagnosed with breast cancer, spent her last months desperately trying to please her father. Ellen had spent most of her life trying to gain her father's approval, and her illness only intensified the quest. Rather than focusing on what she wanted to create, Ellen dedicated herself to manipulating her father, trying to force him to recognize her and thereby validate her life. Ellen immersed herself in problem solving. She was certain she could fix all of her problems by winning her father's recognition. Ellen's "solution" depended on something outside herself that ultimately she could not control—her father's opinion of her.

Of course many factors influence someone's recovery from cancer or any other major illness. I could not definitively say that Ellen's problem-solving orientation was the sole reason for the rapid progression of her disease. Someone struggling with a terminal illness, however, has a greater chance of recovery if she chooses health in order to serve her life visions. The process of creating is essentially a life-affirming pursuit. Creating engages our life force, our innate regenerative capacity, as we birth new projects, objects, or states of being into the world. This creative focus seems to revive the body's generative abilities as well. We can cocreate health in tandem with the realization of our passions and life visions. Choosing health does not guarantee recovery, but choosing health in order to create what matters most can improve the chances of survival.

What Do You Really Want?

If you have a terminal illness, you may argue that you can never have vibrant health, so why should you bother choosing it? Part of the choosing process is to tell yourself the truth about what you really want. Even if you never achieve full health, at least you do not have the additional burden of lying to yourself about what matters most to you. You can tell yourself the truth about what you want and choose health regardless of whether or not you can realize this vision.

Simply choosing health does not guarantee you will achieve health. You will not know until you take action whether or not you can achieve optimal health. Choosing health, however, increases your ability to take appropriate action, evaluate your progress, and adjust your actions as necessary.

Oscillating Structures: The "Yo-Yo" Syndrome

Health strategies designed to minimize risks or circumvent disease soon lose momentum. Any improvement in health diminishes the reason to continue the program: "Hey, my blood pressure is down!" says Joan. "The doctor says I've lowered my risk for heart disease. I'm more relaxed, not so scared anymore so why should I keep up this walking program?"

If avoidance is the motivation for taking action, the greater the distance from the feared event, the less reason you have to take action. In the avoidance strategy, the closer you are to the feared event (for example, illness, stroke, death, severe pain), the more action you will take. As soon as health improves, however, the impetus to take action diminishes.

After lapsing into her old ways, Joan's blood pressure probably will rise again. The pounds she struggled so hard to lose will return . . .plus a few more. As Joan's health deteriorates, the desire to improve her health increases. She "motivates" herself and returns to her healthy diet and exercise program.

This familiar pattern of yo-yoing toward and away from your desired goals is what Robert Fritz, author of *The Path of Least Resistance*, calls an "oscillating structure."[1] Joan truly wants good health. She also really wants to eat rich food and avoid exercise. These two goals are in conflict. Joan can't have *both* health *and* an overly rich diet and no exercise.

Imagine this woman standing between her two opposite desires—health on one side and her favorite foods and lack of exercise on the other. Imagine a rubber band connecting her to health, and another rubber band connecting her to her beloved foods and her easy chair. The conflict generates a pendulum-like series of actions for the would-be health enthusiast. As soon as she moves toward "health," the pull toward the opposite desire becomes stronger. She overcomes the opposite pull by "motivating" herself, pumping herself up with books, audiocassettes, and declarations to all of her friends about her goals. The closer she moves to health, however, the stronger the pull toward her beloved foods and comfortable chair. When she follows the stronger pull, abandoning her exercise program and resuming her usual diet, the pull toward health will be stronger. She resolves to "try harder," buys several new books and a video for motivation, and begins yet another swing in the direction of health. She will choose one goal or the other, depending on where she is in the oscillating structure.

Many patients are mystified when they return to their former habits, regain weight, stop exercising, and feel fatigued. No amount of motivation, inspiration, or perspiration will propel you toward your vision of health if you are focused on preventing disease. Choosing health is a vital step toward the creation of health, yet any attempt to "fix" an oscillating structure by choosing health only reinforces the oscillation. Unfortunately we cannot problem-solve our way out of an oscillating structure. For someone swinging back and forth, choosing health may be yet another attempt at fixing, resolving, or altering the oscillating structure. Within a resolving structure, however, the choice to create health catalyzes the fulfillment of your vision.

The "Do-or-Die" Syndrome

Many people in an oscillating structure will abandon their health goals at the first "transgression." "Darn," says the woman in the oscillating structure, devouring hot fudge and ice cream. "I thought I was going to make it this time. I told myself this was it, do or die. I was going to lower my blood pressure or else! Well, I've blown it now. All that good work, and now I'm eating this hot-fudge sundae. Sigh. I might as well order a steak and some fries and a milkshake. What the heck—I've blown it already, right? I think I'll make reservations for Bob's Super Pig-Out Buffet tomorrow night. I mean, I haven't eaten there for at least a month!"

Resolving Structures: Moving toward Your Goals

Someone who has chosen to be healthy may take the very same actions as a health enthusiast operating in the avoidance strategy. The person who has chosen health, however, is moving toward a desired outcome rather than away from what she fears. When health improves, she will continue walking, even though her cholesterol levels have dropped. She will continue eating healthy food, even though her triglyceride levels have returned to normal. "I feel great!" she proclaims. "I want to feel this way when I'm seventy-five, so I'm keeping up my walking program and eating healthy food. I haven't felt this good since I was sixteen!"

Robert Fritz describes this movement as a "resolving structure." Here the person is not oscillating between two opposite goals. Instead, she has *chosen* her vision of health and is making choices to support the realization of that vision. Sure, she may still love hot-fudge sundaes and sitting for hours in front of the TV watching her favorite sit-coms. Her choice for health, however, creates a hierarchy for her decisions. She may *want* to eat the hot-fudge sundae, but she chooses an apple instead. She doesn't pretend she doesn't love ice cream, but rather makes a choice *for* what she wants. "Ooooh," she says to herself. "That hot-fudge sundae looks *so* good. I *love* the way the hot fudge softens the top of the ice cream, and those crunchy nuts, and the way the whipped cream melts in my mouth . . .yeah, and here's the apple in the fridge. Yep, I'm choosing the apple. I've decided to keep my cholesterol down, so it's apples for me."

If this woman does choose at some point to eat a hot-fudge sundae or a pile of fried chicken, gravy, and biscuits smothered with butter, she most likely will resume her healthy eating habits. The grease binge is a temporary deviation, not a complete oscillation in her journey toward health. She stuffs herself at the family reunion and spends the day lolling around in the shade, visiting with family. The next day, however, she resumes her exercise program and healthy diet. She still desires health and continues making choices for her health, despite the temporary detour. Her choice is for a lifetime, not just a short-term goal such as lowering her cholesterol levels.

CREATE A CLEAR PICTURE OF HEALTH

What does health look like to you? Do you have an image of yourself in full, vibrant health? Take a few minutes to compose a clear picture for yourself (either mentally or on paper). Sketch in as much detail as possible. Paint the picture as completely and boldly as you can. For right now, forget about whether or not your picture is "realistic." Many of the great innovations of our time would never have been completed if their creators had insisted on being "realistic." Just tell yourself the truth about how you want to look, how you want to feel, and what a healthy life looks like for you. Include all the elements of health— physical, mental, emotional, spiritual, and environmental—that are important to you. As you create this picture, ask yourself the following questions:

1. "Have I told myself the truth about what I really want?"
   For the moment, forget about what you think is possible. Just tell yourself the unedited truth about what you want. You may want to lose every ounce of cellulite on your thighs and buttocks but hesitate to include that detail in the vision for a variety of reasons. You sigh and say, "I've had jiggling, chubby thighs since I was four years old—

that will never change." The fact that you've always had chubby thighs does not change your desire to have firm thighs. Be honest with yourself about what you really want.

2. "Have I diminished the vision so that I'm more comfortable with it?"
   Diminishing your goals may make you feel more comfortable in the short term—"Phew, I'm not as far away as I thought!"—but in the long run you lose the full power of your original vision.

3. "Do I have specific goals that I would recognize if I reached them?"
   Create a vision that you can accurately measure. Each aspect of the vision will have its own standard of measurement. "Weigh 130 pounds," for example, is a very different vision from "Have 19 percent body fat." The first vision requires a scale. The second calls for a body-composition machine or underwater test to determine the percentage of body fat. You will know if you have a vague goal if you cannot find a good standard of measurement. "Lose some weight" or "Bring down my blood pressure" are not specific goals. How much is "some" weight? Two pounds? Two hundred pounds? Does "bringing down" blood pressure mean diastolic or systolic blood pressure (the upper and lower numbers)? Both? How much do you want to reduce blood pressure? "Consistent blood pressure readings of 120/80 for a month" is a much more specific vision with a clearly defined measurement.

4. "If I could inhabit this vision, would I take it?"
   This question reminds you to fill in any details or discard any extraneous elements in your vision. Maybe you discover that your desire for a twenty-six-inch waist was the result of your brother's incessant childhood teasing. Is that what you really want now? If the answer is "Yes!" by all means include it in the vision. If not, discard that detail. Maybe life just isn't worth living unless you have a garden or live near the ocean. Make sure you include all of the elements of health that are important to you.

5. "Do I choose to be healthy?"
   Remember the power of choosing health.

Know Where You Are in Relationship to Your Vision

As with any journey, you need a good idea of where you are before you begin. Imagine wanting to drive from Los Angeles to New York City but telling yourself you are in Seattle, Washington. If you start making decisions as if you were in Seattle, you have very little chance of reaching New York.

Where are you now? What is your state of health? Answer that question as accurately and completely as possible. You may choose to have an annual physical to measure the basics, for example, blood pressure, reflexes, blood work, and a Pap smear for women. In addition, gather information about your current lifestyle—what are you eating, how much are you exercising, how much stress you have in your life, and how effectively you are coping with that stress. Use the questionnaires and charts at the end of this chapter to help you create an accurate picture of where you are now in relation to your health goals.

As you make lifestyle changes, the current health picture will change. You will need to reassess your state of health as you progress. Having an accurate picture of your current state helps you to choose appropriate next steps.

For the next week, keep track of your diet and exercise using the diet diary and exercise journal below. You will find additional copies of the diet diary and exercise journal at the end of the book. You are welcome to photocopy these charts so that you can use them again and again to get an accurate read on your current state of health.

Types of Exercise

There are four main types of exercise for you to keep track of:

1. **Aerobic exercise**: Rhythmic, continuous exercise using the large muscles of the body (legs) that deepens breathing and increases the heartbeat to target heart rate (for how to calculate target heart rate, see p. XX). Examples: Walking, jogging, running, swimming, rowing.

2. **Strength-building exercise**: Resistance exercise that increases muscle strength. Examples: Isometrics, calisthenics, weight lifting, sprinting, some yoga postures.

3. **Stretching exercise**: Stretching and holding muscles at just less than the point of discomfort. Example: Yoga.

Diet Diary for _____ **Beginning Date** _____

The purpose of this diary is to provide you and your doctor with an unbiased record of your normal eating habits. Simply eat your typical diet and record what you eat for seven days in succession. Under breakfast, lunch, and dinner columns list food and drink ingredients and amounts. Under BM, list bowel movement times. Under Notes, list symptoms such as mood swings, indigestion, headaches, fatigue, and so on. Remember to include snacks and supplements (brand name, ingredients, potency).

	SUNDAY	MONDAY	TUESDAY	WEDNESDAY	THURSDAY	FRIDAY	SATURDAY
BREAKFAST							
LUNCH							
DINNER							
BM TIMES							

Additional Notes:

Exercise Journal for _____ Beginning Date _____

The purpose of this diary is to provide you and your doctor with an unbiased record of your normal exercise habits. Simply follow your typical exercise routine and record what you do for seven days in sucession. For every day list the amount and type of exercise you do.

   * Note any physical, mental, or emotional responses to exercise, such as muscle strains after certain kinds of exercise, enjoyment or dislike of particular types of exercise, and so on.

	SUNDAY	MONDAY	TUESDAY	WEDNESDAY	THURSDAY	FRIDAY	SATURDAY
AEROBIC							
STRENGTH-BUILDING							
STRETCHING							
ACTIVITIES OF DAILY LIVING							
RESPONSES TO EXERCISE*							

Additional Notes:

4. **Activities of Daily Living (ADL)**: Activities at work or at home that require movement. Examples: Typing, vacuuming, gardening, driving, doing laundry.

In addition to reviewing your diet and exercise habits, I also highly recommend getting a copy of *The Stress Map*. This invaluable tool allows you to assess four aspects of stress in your life: your environment (work and personal), coping responses, inner world (thoughts and feelings), and signals of distress. The last section offers suggestions to address specific areas of "strain" or "burnout." Photocopy the "map" in the center so that you can reuse it in the future. You can order *The Stress Map* at your local bookstore or directly from Newmarket Press.[2]

Work with Structural Tension

The disparity between your current state and the place you want to be generates a tension that moves you toward your destination. In his book *The Path of Least Resistance*, Robert Fritz calls this "structural tension." Think of the anticipation at the beginning of a road trip. You have packed the car, studied the road map, and chosen your route. Finally you turn on the ignition and roll down the driveway. You imagine the skyscrapers of New York and that final drive across one of the bridges onto the island of Manhattan. For the moment, you are aware of the hot, hazy skies and palm-lined boulevards of Los Angeles.

The difference between your current location and your final destination creates a tension. Imagine a huge rubber band stretching across the continent, connecting your car in Los Angeles with your desired destination in New York. On a road trip, you may experience this tension as "anticipation." A painter may recognize this tension as a sense of urgency or increased focus on her work. All creators recognize this pull between their desired creation and their current situation. As a creator of health, you may recognize this "tension" as a powerful force that propels you toward your desired vision of health. You can maintain this structural tension by accurately observing your current state while simultaneously holding an image of your desired state of health.

Vision Develops Organically

Some people have a hard time envisioning what they have never experienced. If you have never known vibrant health, how can you envision yourself as healthy? Developing a vision for health may be an ongoing process. Consider the development of a baby in the womb. Imagine being pregnant but not knowing exactly what the baby will look like. You may not even know if the baby is a girl or a boy. As the baby develops, you can feel movement inside. Eventually you can trace the outlines of the baby's limb poking against your belly; you begin to know its shape. Not until the baby is born, however, will you know all of the details of this newly emerging being.

The creation process inherently involves mystery. We can't know every step of the process in advance. The seed of vision grows within us. We nourish that seed with deliberate choices, "fortuitous" meetings, and unexpected intuitions.

The Journey to Health

You will be using the following chart throughout the book to assess your current location and your vision of health (desired destination). After much thought, I carefully chose the word "journey" to describe this exploration of health. A "map" or "path" implies an already established course and a known destination. A journey, however, may require forging a completely new route. Your journey to health will be unique to you, shaped by your personal vision of health. Perhaps you will follow established pathways to create your vision of health. Your vision may require you to bushwhack into unknown territory or to combine the known and unknown byways. I cannot offer a predetermined pathway with a guaranteed destination. Your own vision of health has more power, truth, and passion than any ready-made, one-size-fits-all program I could present to you. Instead, I offer tools to assist you in navigating on your own journey to health.

Complete the journey to health chart in seven steps:

1. Describe your destination (the state of health you desire).

2. Accurately describe your current location (your current state of health).

3. Notice the difference between where you are and where you want to be.

4. Ask yourself, "If I could have my desired state of health, would I take it?"

Vision: desired state of health

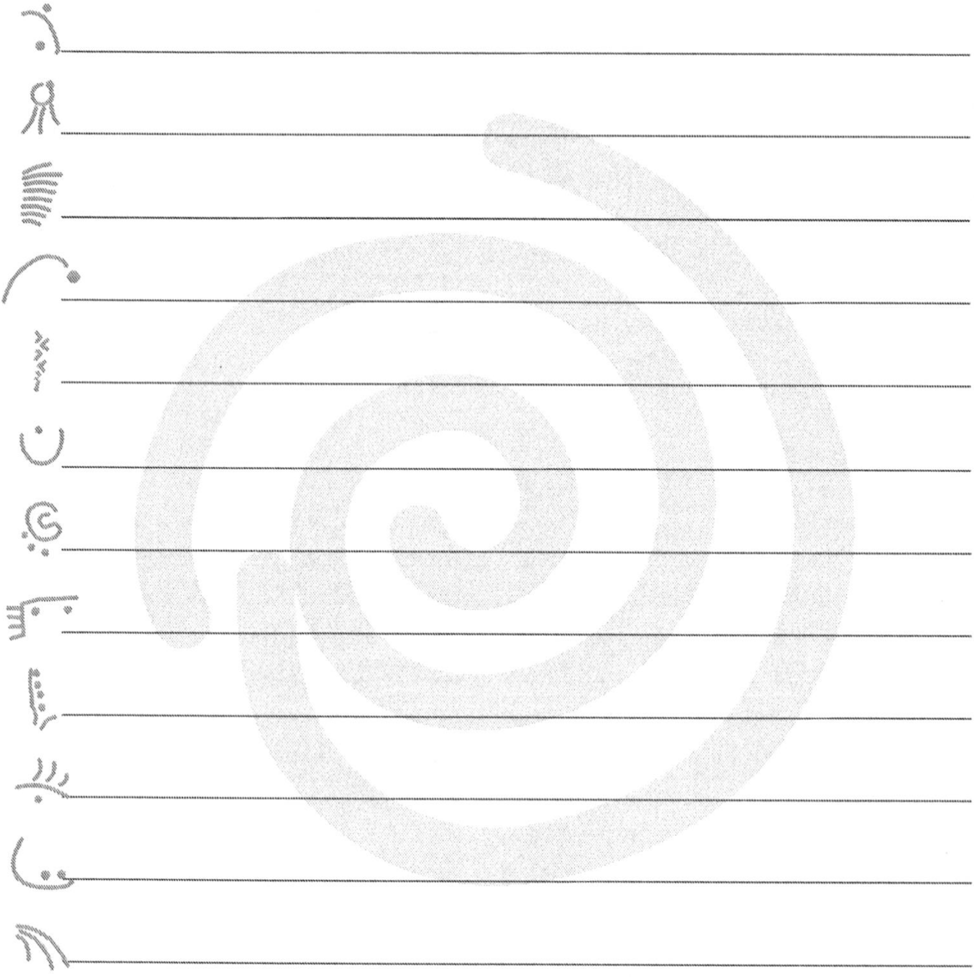

_____

_____

_____

_____

_____

_____

_____

_____

_____

_____

_____

Current location: present state of health

see options for this chart in options.pdf

5. If the answer is "Yes," then CHOOSE that state of health. "I choose . . ." and describe what you desire.

6. Simultaneously hold an image of your desired state and your current state of health. Notice the structural tension generated by the disparity between the two pictures.

7. Fill in action steps that will move you toward your destination.

Make choices that support your vision of health

As soon as you have a clear destination and a well-defined current location, think of steps you can take to fulfill your vision. These steps are secondary choices that support your primary choice to be healthy (see below for examples of specific steps). Write down as many steps as occur to you. These action steps arise from reviewing your final destination, clarifying your current position, and then defining the discrepancy between the two locations.

Create, Evaluate, and Adjust

Keep in mind that you will be adjusting these secondary choices over time as you progress on your journey toward health. You may discover, for example, a particular exercise program that better fits your goals than the exercise you have been doing. After beginning the new program, evaluate the effect of your actions. Has the exercise program moved you toward your vision? Has your health improved as a result of the program? How has your health improved? Remember the importance of having accurate measurements (for example, blood pressure readings, body composition tests, or energy levels) to determine the effectiveness of your actions. The action steps are flexible, subject to evaluation and adjustment. New steps will occur to you as you continue on the journey toward health.

Following the Yellow Brick Road: Evaluating Your Action Steps

As you create your action steps, ask yourself the following questions:

◆ Will this action step move me toward my vision of health? What part of my vision?

Vision of health

Colleen wants to reduce her blood pressure, and decides that her goal is a consistent reading of 125/80 for a month. She also wants to have sex with her partner twice a week. Colleen wants enough energy to get through the day at work and then come home to work in the garden during the spring and summer and paint (watercolor) during the winter.

Action steps on the road to health

Practice with deep relaxation tape five times a week. Complete by _____

Eliminate coffee. Complete by _____

Eat black beans for breakfast. Complete by _____

Exercise at lunchtime and during breaks for a total of thirty minutes per day. Complete by _____

Take public transportation to work. (increases reading time, reduces stress of rush-hour commute) Complete _____

Practice good sleep hygiene. Complete by _____

Eliminate simple carbohydrates. Complete by _____

Eat three servings of whole grains per day. Complete by _____

Eliminate red meat. Complete by _____

Eat fish three times a week. Complete by _____

15 percent body fat. Complete by _____

Schedule "dates" to make love with my partner when we are not tired or stressed. Complete by _____

Current health

At her last doctor's visit two months ago, fifty-six-year-old Colleen's blood pressure was 165/95. She periodically checks her own blood pressure and averages about 160/95. Her body composition is 29 percent fat. For the last six months, Colleen has been too tired to think about making love. She falls into bed exhausted at 9 p.m. but can't fall asleep until 11 p.m. She sleeps fitfully and gets up at least twice during the night to pee. She gets out of bed at 6 a.m. and jump-starts the coffeemaker. Armed with a large mug of coffee and a pastry, she leaves the house at 6:30 a.m. and spends an hour on the congested freeway driving to work. She grinds through the day attending meetings, answering phone calls, and doing paper work. At noon, she eats a pepperoni pizza and a cola delivered by a nearby pizza parlor. By 3 p.m. she barely can keep her eyes open, despite having drunk eight cups of coffee. At 4:30 p.m. she leaves the office and spends ninety minutes driving through rush-hour traffic. When she arrives home at 6 p.m., she looks at the overgrown garden, groans and retreats to the sofa for an hour's nap. She wakes at 7 p.m., greets her partner, and sits down to a big pasta dinner. She watches a couple of TV shows. At 9 p.m., too sleepy to watch the next show, Colleen crawls into bed and lies staring at the ceiling until she finally falls asleep around 11 p.m.

- Is the action step specific enough? Do I have an accurate way of measuring the results?

- Will I recognize the result when I see it?

- Have I specified a date by which I will complete this step? Having a specific date helps you organize your actions. If Colleen decided to reduce body fat to 20 percent in five years, she would take different actions than if she decided to complete that step in twelve months.

- Which action step is most important right now? Choose the most important action steps first. Someone with diabetes, for example, might focus first on reducing and stabilizing blood sugar levels by eliminating simple sugars, increasing beans in the diet, and supplementing chromium.

Where Am I Going Next? (Always Have a Place to Go.)

Chapters 9, 10, and 11 (nutrition and exercise) will assist you in refining your action steps. The exercises you have completed in this chapter provide both an accurate description of your current state of health *and* an accurate baseline by which to assess your progress. As you embark on this new journey, you probably have lots of questions: What will I eat? Will the terrain be friendly? Will I have companions along the way? Stay tuned for more secrets to help make your journey a success.

Exercise Adherence Questionnaire

This series of questions is intended to help you discover your attitudes, prejudices, and preferences about exercise. Consider the questions fuel for thought to help you discover the type of exercise that best suits you.

DIRECTIONS

Check each statement that applies to you. If you have additional beliefs you'd like to add, please write them on the blank lines.

Beliefs

- ❑ I am too old to exercise.

- ❑ Exercise only helps if you do a lot, and I'm not an iron man!

❑ I think I am uncoordinated and feel too embarrassed to exercise.

❑ Exercise is all work and no play.

❑ I will be injured if I begin to exercise.

❑ Sweating is disgusting.

❑ Exercise is good for my health.

My Style

❑ I drive myself hard.

❑ If something seems too hard, I will give up.

❑ I prefer to exercise alone.

❑ I love team sports.

❑ I would exercise more consistently if I worked out with a group or a friend.

❑ I want immediate results or I will not stick to my program.

❑ When I relapse from my exercise program due to injury or illness:

   ❑ I probably won't start again.

   ❑ I will ridicule myself for stopping my exercise program.

   ❑ I will certainly begin exercising again.

❑ _____

MY SUPPORT TEAM

❑ The people I live with think exercise is silly.

❑ Even though no one at home supports my exercise program, I have a friend or family member who will.

❑ The people I live with will be neutral about my exercise program.

❑ The people I live with will be encouraging of my exercise program.

❑ I care what other people think of me.

❑ I don't give a hoot about what others think.

MY CHOICES

❑ I have chosen to exercise to support my vision of health.

❑ I *can't* exercise now . . . maybe later.

❑ Not now, not ever!

MY HISTORY

❑ I was usually the last one picked for school teams.

❑ I have been made fun of while playing sports or wearing a bathing suit.

❑ I was a super jock in high school or college.

❑ Moderate exercise has always been part of my daily life.

Historical/Cultural Background

Today the Iroquois are a league of six nations of eastern aboriginal First Peoples on this continent currently called North America. Their cultural-political paradigm is the world's oldest, purest, still functioning democracy; it also happens to be a matriarchy.

To the Iroquois scholar, the notion that democracy began in Greece is like a bad "knock-knock" joke as the version of "democracy" practiced in ancient Greece was more "hypocrisy!" The Greeks enslaved two-thirds of their population, and never granted women and children equality. Unlike all other democracies, all the citizens of the matriarchal Iroquois League of Nations were and are so well represented that the men, the old people, and the children are equally as happy and content as the women!

The Iroquois embrace certain irrefutable precepts—one of them being the autonomy of women. This is, after all, a female planet—*the Mother Earth*—and, as such, a woman's "place" is "wherever she wants to be."

Reflections by AmyLee

Buweh's Daughter, AmyLee, is the last in her lineage of Medicine Women. Born to Iroquois parents, AmyLee spent the first twenty-one years of her life studying and serving her Grandmother's "medicine-way practice." Graduating from her apprenticeship as a Medicine Woman Initiate, AmyLee continued her medicine journey by studying with and serving other Elders. A part of that next twenty-one-year-long initiation involved guiding the many women whose own power they recognized, mirrored by hers.

In 1970, AmyLee cofounded the American Indian Rights Association, which in 1985 evolved into the present-day Native American Indian Resource Center, Inc.

As Gate-Keeper to the Star Sisterhood of the Dancing Shields, AmyLee has written to, spoken with, ceremonied for, and otherwise gifted that emerging circle of amazing women for over eighteen years.

The little girl Yehauweh had been asked the same question often, and her reply was always the same. And her answer became her affirmation, easily attested to by the jut of her chin and her firmly planted feet. In her voice, there was an unmistakable air of pride married with patient anticipation.

"What do I want to be when I grow older? I want to be an Old Woman!"

To those from cultures other than hers, her aspiration caused unease, even nervous laughter.

To those of her Haudenesaunee (Iroquois) culture, her smile was mirrored on their knowing faces.

This Daughter of the Haudenesaunee is proud to have been born all that she is, proud of what she will one day become, which hopefully in time will include becoming an Old Woman.

It is the night following her day-long Becoming a Woman Celebration. And what a celebration it was!

All her Aunties and Sisters, her Mother's and hers, and even Clan Mothers from other Families had come just to honor her!

Yehauweh scrunched deeper into her fur-covered bed near the floor. Filled with cattail down and fresh cedar fronds, then covered in thin white doeskin and layered in fur pelts her Uncles had given her, her bed was soft and wonderful. She wriggled and rolled as she slept, tossing dreams and memories about like popping corn.

There were so many memories of the celebration!

"Her Day" began with a bath of "smell 'ums"—those precious herbs that always made her tingle and sneeze and that made her whole body feel as if it was inhaling a rush of fresh air. The Old Women brushed her wet hair with smell 'ums too. While Yehuaweh lay covered in her small drying blanket, they tickled her lovingly and patted her all over. They told her jokes she would someday laugh at. Together they savored sweet teas and corncakes and smashed berries with maple sugar. Songs were sung. Rows of little and big bundles sat nearby on a bench, and they were all for her!

Each of the Aunties in attendance had offered her some piece of wisdom for becoming a woman on this female planet. Her eyes and ears took everything in, holding it safe in her heart and mind.

One of her Aunties told her, "The true powers of this planet, and of each person, are in the *balance* between the Right Hand and the Left Hand." (She remembered the stories she had heard told every year ever since she could remember, the stories about the Left-Handed and Right-Handed Twins. The story her Auntie told now seemed to be their sequel.)

"There is nothing 'good' about one and 'bad' about the other side, the other twin. It is in the imbalance that the problems begin. People today speak of 'positive' as being 'good' and 'negative' as being 'bad.' That out-of-balance way of looking at the world began the last time the prominence on this earth slipped away from women's care and back into men's care.

"It wasn't one of our best moments in history. Perhaps we women were reluctant to release that prominence (what some would misinterpret as a right to dominance). Perhaps the men were too eager to claim it, ripping it away from us with force and maligning all that is woman."

The Aunties paused here. Though they had shown Yehauweh this before, they once again showed her how her female body was made of thirteen spaces that were all connected and how the energy they emitted swirled first inside of her and then outside of her, like rings of a tree but stacked upright instead of around. Each ring moved in the opposite direction. She was female, which meant seven of her "rings" swirled counterclockwise while six swirled clockwise. Her cousin, a boy, would be the opposite. His seven rings swirled clockwise and the other six counterclockwise. And in the sum total of it all, those rings held them together. They made her a little girl becoming woman and made him a little boy becoming man. Those rings that ran clockwise like rivers of energy were held by the Right-Hand Twin and were called "positive" by some. Positive was good. It always has been. The rings under the custody of the Left-Hand Twin swirled counterclockwise and were called "negative." Negative was good. It always has been.

"Positive is good and is the daylight, guarded by the Grandfather Sun and Father Sky. Negative is good and is the nighttime, guarded by the Grandmother Moon, the Star Women, and the Mother Earth," another Auntied continued. "When the people forgot, or pretended to forget, that women were as "good" as men, that negative was as "good" as positive, that the night was as "good" as the day, then the balance was upset and calamity ensued."

One of the Aunties had gone away to college, and she spoke many languages: that of her people, the Seneca, and that of her neighbors, English, and that of the college, Science.

"Just as we have always known that the world is comprised of the balance between the Left Hand and the Right Hand, the Night and the Day, the Moon and the Sun, the Women and the Men," she said, "the Academicians are learning that fact too, in their own way, in their own time. They now talk about positive and negative parts of each atom and the tension between the two as being that which holds all matter together. They have yet to realize that the dance goes far beyond the microscope—and that both the negative and positive are good, are equal in importance."

Another Old Auntie added, "When a woman forgets that negative is good, and that it is the imbalance between negative and positive that makes the problems, then she has disowned $7/13$ths of herself, more than half of herself! She has said to herself, her Sisters, her Elders, her Children, and to all Men, that she is the cause of all things bad. She has insulted the Moon and the Sun, for they love and respect one another. When one takes a hit, the other falls too."

They were on a roll now. A room full of Aunties sparked off one another in rapid-fire sequence. "Yes, Sister, you are right," is how they each began, then added their own round.

"Yes, Sister, you are right. And how would the world be if it were all positive? Only sunshine and no cool shade? Only daylight and no night sleep and dreams? Only smiles pasted on the faces of women who could then not show any other emotion?" (Little did the Auntie know she was prophesying an era of Botox, plastic surgery, and antidepressants that would quell the righteous anger and grief of women who had been denied their potency and prominence.)

The water drum had begun its cadence. There was flute music way off at the edge of the forest. She imagined that the flute music was for her too—perhaps it was being played by that boy from the Deer Clan, wanting to honor her from a respectful distance. Maybe the tangle of wilting wildflowers at the door-stoop had been from him as well. Maybe. (Although, they might have been from her Uncle, who was sad to be losing his best little fishing buddy even for a day.)

While all the directions of the universe converged inside her, as they do inside us each and all, Yehauweh knew that did not mean the world revolved around her even on this very special day. There were prayers and ceremonies and tasks and honors that had little or nothing to do with her, and there were those in which she played an important role by honoring others.

Yehauweh thought back about the weeks and months before her Becoming a Woman Day. For some time, she had been aware of the Old Women noticing her—whispering when she walked away, chortling softly like mama birds to their nested young, hiding whatever they had been working on when she walked back into a room. Old Women were mysterious. She liked that about them. Yehauweh looked forward to having some mysteries of her own someday.

The Aunties also had been observing her, their "Little One," watching her body change and her mind both expand and hone itself. They noted her moods like little tides ebbing on lunar cue.

Yehauweh herself had been noticing some interesting alterations in the landscape of her little body. There was a patch of fine soft "grasses" springing on the slope beneath her lower torso, and small mounds were pushing out the "pink spots" on her chest, and, well, there were other developments too, but she had stayed too busy to notice.

It seemed her life was speeding up, in a race headed somewhere she could not yet see.

And then, she saw.

And her Mother and Grandmothers and Aunties were there to greet and welcome her.

And that brings us back to this fine day—Yehauweh's day, She had rustled through her little cache of belongings, plucking out all but two to give away. It was a sour-sweet parting, as she could have still enjoyed most of those toys, and she had always taken good care of them. However, she was making room for new belongings—and there they sat, wrapped in pretty pale calico cloth, tied in ribbons that she could hardly wait to braid into something fine— maybe even new fishing lures!

After the feasting, and after the speeches and orations and Welcome Dance, and during the songs which changed but never stopped, she sat inside her circle, surrounded by a wheel of gifts to open. Each one's opening brought a cooing and purring and up-and-down nodding from the women who had made a circle around hers. There were baskets, and needles and spools of sinew to sew with, and a tiny mirror with a song about it being "just the right size to see all that's important—anything bigger would just be vanity and a waste of time."

It was these memories that kept popping into her sleep this special night. At last, they all melded into a sweeping swirl of a sweet calm dream.

The night was old when her Mother gently shook Yehauweh's fur-hidden shoulder.

"Yehauweh, Yehauweh, Daughter. It is time to get up. Come."

A wriggle under the blankets. First, a shock of tossled hair emerged, followed by the sleepy face of a blinking Daughter. "Hmmgh? Momma?"

"Come now. Slip your moccasins on. It's time to get up. Your Aunties are waiting for you. They have precious gifts to bestow."

Yehauweh thought for sure she was weaving fresh memory with deep dreams just as she had been dream-weaving all those bright ribbons in her sleep a moment ago.

She laughed at how three-dimensional it all was. "Am I dreaming you?" Her laughter trailed to her Mother, standing beside her.

"No, Daughter, Sister, Friend. It's time." And she guided the Little-One-Becoming-A-Woman, wrapping her new robe around her young-strong shoulders.

As they stood on the threshold, the smoky heat of the longhouse embraced them from behind, then quickly slipped past them out into the darkness. It left its path of blurry white warmth meeting cool night, and they followed.

The sky was the same dark blue of a newborn's eyes. The stars were like popping corn—OK, maybe she was still dreaming! But as the earth met her moccasins, and the twisting breeze filled her nostrils with the damp smells one only knows by night, her other senses fully awakened.

"Momma! Where are we going? It's late!"

Her Mother motioned the sign to hush and just follow. Then the sign to listen, not just with your ears, but your whole body—let the sounds bounce off your bones, ripple across your flesh, tickle your hair and lips. She listened. With her whole being, she listened, and she followed the blanket which was her Mother, striding before her.

That night her Aunties in the woods offered many gifts. The mother Deer and her Fawn bestowed the tandem gifts of Alertness with Tranquility, as the Deer peacefully watched Yehauweh's approach before darting away with her Fawn.

The Bear and her Cub taught Yehauweh of Strength and Love. "Your Auntie the Bear has given you her best gift tonight," explained her mother. "She walks this Turtle Island as the biggest mammal among us. She carries the most power and strength. And her heart, too, is the hugest here. Her gift is the reminder that the most powerful must travel with the biggest heart lest that power be misused. And the biggest heart must be protected by the mightiest strength, lest that heart be broken beyond repair."

Two old Rabbits, Great-Great-Aunties, gifted Yehauweh with the reminder to Play. In the moss, through the ferns, they rolled and hopped and bounced and nibbled.

From nowhere but blackness, and on silent wings that made nothing but swift breeze, Owl swooped in and out again, with one of the Rabbits in her clutches. Yehauweh watched in horror. She didn't know why, she only knew she wanted to cry and hide inside her Mother's robe.

"Yehauweh, your Auntie the Owl has a gift for you this night too."

Yehauweh lifted just one eye above the blanket and sputtered, "I don't want it."

Finally, after many tears, Yehauweh emerged from her Mother's wool blanket.

"What is it? The gift."

"Your Auntie the Owl lets herself be misunderstood. She is that strong! And powerful. So strong is she that when confused people fear her, or tell stories and jokes about her, she just waits and watches. She comes into our lives on silent wings, with a haunting cry, to let us know she is there, and willing. She is willing to take away all our confusion—our misunderstandings, our projections, and she will carry them away to be transformed in her flight. It does not hurt nor harm her. She does this willingly, lovingly, not just for us but so that we might walk more tenderly on the earth and thus treat all life more kindly, without the pain of fear, of confusion."

And they began their journey home.

With the silhouette of the longhouse in dim sight, they paused to look over their shoulders. It had been the longest short walk they had ever shared. It was then they heard the howling. It came from the ledge beyond the fir, under the Moon, near the horizon.

Otyoneh, the Wolf, offered her gift.

"Yehauweh. How did we go away and come home?"

"We followed the paths we always take."

Her Mother nodded, "Ah huh. And the paths we followed were made by whom?"

"By us, I guess."

"Ummmm. And how did we know where to make those paths?"

She thought back to the generations of her family who had called this woods "home," and how it was possible to live here that long, and then she got it! "The Deer and the Bear and the Rabbits made the paths first—and we followed so we could eat, and have clothes, and medicine and tools and…" She looked to her Mother-Teacher for confirmation.

"Ummm. And how did all those animals and others know where to make their paths and trails?"

"Momma, that's too hard. I wasn't even here then." Oytoneh howled in the distance. Her mother turned her head toward the howl of Oytoneh.

"You mean her? My Wolf Auntie? Why would anybody follow a Wolf! Why wouldn't they be going the other way—and fast!"

Her Mother chuckled then continued, "Yehauweh, your Auntie the Wolf is the Trailblazer. All the roads and highways of Humans began as animal trails and paths. And before that, they were the faint foot marks from the padded feet of Wolves, as they led themselves and all others to the safe sources of drinking water. Tonight she watched over us as we made our way along her path and back again. She has instilled in you her gift for making trails and following them safely."

"Wow." Yehauweh didn't know which way to step next for fear she'd make a mistake and insult her Auntie. So she just held still, still—until a tiny aching howl moved through her body, blazing its way into her consciousness. When it reached her feet, they moved. And they carried her around to the front of the lodge.

There Grandmother Moon awaited them. Just as her Mother was about to say something—something wise, no doubt—they tripped over the same stone and toppled onto one another on their way to the ground!

"Oh my!" Mother cried.

"Oh my!" Yehauweh echoed her Mother.

Laughing, they sat back on their elbows and looked up, down, and all around.

One of these wise Daughters spoke, "Well, there is no better place to fall than onto the waiting breast of our Earth Mother!"

And the other wise Daughter added, "And there is no better view of our Moon Grandmother as she smiles on us!"

Yehauweh would fall often. And just as often, she would look up to the Moon and down to the Earth and smile. She had become a good Woman on this female planet. Her works spoke for her heart. The trail behind her was made smoother for those who followed. And those along the way had been blessed and bettered for having known her kindness and example.

Yehauweh called a Daughter to be born through her. A Sister. A Friend.

Together they embraced the rainbow of experiences only a mother and daughter can know. There was love—and anger. There was laughter—and stinging tears. There were battles that no one would win, and those that no one really wanted to win. And through it all, the love endured, the love that was an unbreakable promise to "be there" for one another, to the best of their ability to be so, and to forgive the times they weren't—and to not stop loving for hurdles such as anger, distraction, or death. Some loves are eternal. And some loves are even better after at least one of the Beloveds has traveled the Starry Road to the next life, leaving behind all the burden baskets of ego and desire.

It is then that only love remains, and follows, and returns...

Many years later, as the frost coated Yehauweh's raven black hair, she got a bigger mirror. And that is where she spent her ration of vanity and time. Lady Clairol covered her secrets for her, the same way Playtex hugged her so hard around the middle that no one else could get close.

It was a new era for Indians. For women. For Yehauweh.

New things are often confusing and don't become settled until they are old.

But that didn't stop Yehauweh from sporting the newness of the era to which she was born. Instead of going to her Mother, the Medicine Woman, for herbs, she went to the newly approved AMA white male doctor for a prescription. She felt proud of her modern, "enlightened" choices, as they were confirmed by so many more people—people in magazines and on television, and at work and the new neighbors next door and her new lover and . . .everybody new and confusing in her life.

The Old Ones just watched, and then, one by one, they faded away.

Her Mother, the Medicine Woman for so many and from as many walks of life, kept the herbs handy. It was hard to watch her Daughter bleed too much, bend over in cramps, sweat and shiver, then grumble. It wasn't any easier being snapped at by her tongue like a tightly strung bow let loose. Perhaps it was hardest to bypass her own Daughter, and hand the Medicine over to her Daughter's Daughter, who waited with openness and gratitude. But, alas, that was all part of the lineage prophecy, and they each were living their agreements to it.

Yehauweh alternately felt cherished and chastised—and always outnumbered—when the two generations would squeeze her like the filling in their inescapable sandwich. It felt good to be noticed and loved and fussed over when she wasn't feeling well. It felt embarrassing when the Old Medicine Woman and the young Medicine Girl would say, in chiding unison, "You must be having the world's longest menopause on record—what are you up to now? Nine years? Twelve if you count pouting in self-pity as a symptom?"

She resented their know-it-all tone, partly because they did know it all. And their tone was but a faint echo to the screaming voice of her own knowing. That voice inside echoed, "It will be over when you are ready to get over it, when you are ready to lay it down, dust off your moccasins, and move on." Until then, you can stay jammed in your own doorway, refusing to be budged out into the next phase of your life—but don't expect anybody to visit you until there's room, and they are made comfortable by your own comfort."

She spent a lot of time alone. Just her, and her doorway, and her Lady Clairol, and her Playtex girdle, her little yellow pills in the white envelope, and her too-big mirror in which she refused to see herself.

All the while, the Daughter behind her, and the Mother ahead of her, paced and planned, and scheduled—and then cancelled—so many celebrations for Yehauweh.

"At this rate, I'll be an Elder before my Mother is," the waiting Daughter mumbled to the Moon.

And then it happened, or, rather, "it" didn't! She was done. There would be no more bleeding into the earth or onto the store-bought "sanitary" napkins safety-pinned to her rayon panties and smashed into her Playtex girdle. She was done. With one time in her life now over and ready to begin the next, she took a determined step forward. (Later she would say she had been pushed, but she would then laugh and say the backside of her ego had snapped, along with the elastic in her undergarment. And she'd then turn to her Daughter and mock, "You have something to look forward to." And then one of them would laugh again.)

Yehauweh hadn't really expected much of a party this time, figuring there wasn't really much awaiting her in life, no offense to her Mother who seemed to really be enjoying being an Old Woman . . .and, curiously to Yehauweh, everybody else seemed to be enjoying the Old Woman's oldness too.

But just the same, Yehauweh dressed in her best—girdle. Her beribboned leggings still carried the ribbons of her Becoming a Woman Celebration, with subsequent layers, generations of adornment, embroidered over them. And her over-dress fit pretty good, "for an old lady," she quipped in that too-big mirror. The Tree of Peace medallion hung around her neck, as did rows of meaningful beads. She felt as though all the Elders who had loved her, who had attended her Becoming Ceremony so long ago, were standing with her, placing the strands of their own lives around hers. "I feel like a tree—with a lot of rings." She added the last ring, her beaded moose-hide brow band, around her now white-streaked hair. Looking into the mirror, she was glad it was so big, so she could see the memories, the concentric circles of women who had loved her throughout her past, and when her eyes met her eyes, she saw the Daughter of her Mother, and all the eyes smiled.

She was right. It wasn't much of a party. "Well," her Mother spoke, "you waited until almost everybody was dead. What kind of a turnout did you expect?"

Her young Daughter quipped, "More corn soup for you! You always worried there'd never be enough to go around."

Some "borrowed" Elders from other traditions had come. That was nice—or curious.

They didn't know what to bring, so they brought Jell-O. The table looked real pretty and festive.

The LP played the longhouse music with the added beat of a scratch that made the needle skip.

Everyone decided to move to the smallest room, crowded, but there was no draft there to chill Great-Great-Great-Great-Aunt Sadie.

And the chairs were more comfy too.

Old Women talked about their loves and lives.

After a couple hours, nylon hose were rolled down on their elastic rubber-band-like garters, and legs were casually dangled over the stuffed arms of comfy chairs, and burps could be heard without apology. If a breast or some other part itched, it got scratched. Two sets of false teeth lay together on the mahogany plant stand, as though they were laughing and having a private conversation.

Great-Aunt Bertha leaned over to Elder Cousin Maggie and asked, "What's with Howie? She looks all cinched up and stiff."

The Older One smacked her wrinkly lips and softly chided, "Oh, Yehauweh is still sucking in, holding on, and keeping up…appearances."

"Oh," Bertha knowingly nodded, "she hasn't let it down, let it out, and let it go yet, eh? Too bad. …in time." The soft hammocks of her arms cradled her low slung bosom as her whole body nodded in knowing. Side-by-side the two Old Women wore on their faces all the paths and trails of who they'd been and what they'd done with their lives. Some would call them wrinkles. They called them their "maps."

"Never been lost, not once," they added.

And you'd believe them too.

Jokes of all colors of dirty and clean were bantered and batted about. Yehauweh's cheeks turned the color of cherry Jell-O. In fact, everyone else was laughing so hard that all around the room their little bowls of half-eaten gelatin shook and shimmied like melted-down lava lamps.

As she took it all in with one long sweeping stare, Yehauweh saw there was nothing left to fear. These women were strong—even with a hunched back or a brittle skeleton, toothless, or bespectacled in trifocals—these women where strong, not in spite of their age or infirmities but because of them. There were no victims here. Nobody was taking an ego pity-ride on their hardship, injury or loss. "That's not who I am, what undid me, took me down, that's what made me stronger," one would say.

Old Loves and Old Lives and Old Mothers and Old Wives were swapping the treasures of their time, and through it all, Yehauweh moved from a place of resistance and disdain into a new Freedom . . .a release, like unstringing a bow or . . .ungirdling a woman. She didn't have a word for the taste of it yet, this new freedom. Perhaps she'd have to make one. But this she knew, there was no turning back. And there was no longer a desire to.

Through the ensuing years, Yehauweh grew to embrace that freedom. It wore many names while it danced with her.

Freedom meant doing what she wanted, when she wanted to do it, and feeling good about herself before, during, and after.

Freedom meant acting like a kid if she wanted to, without fear or judgment. Oh, there would still be judges, but, pffff, who were they to expect her to replace her own sense of self with their opinions, projections, ignorance, or arrogance! And some days, she'd be a righteous Old Woman—throw her weight around and put others in the uncomfortable position of having to either honor and respect then tend her needs, or swallow their own embarrassing refusal.

"This Old Woman thing is my ticket," she gleamed. "I cut in front of people in the store. They may think I'm being rude, but hey, I'm an Old Woman, so I just look up at them and smile and say, in my most grandmotherly voice, 'Oh, you're not Indian, are you? We do this for our Elders. Would you carry my bags for me, dear?'"

She spent years, decades really, sashaying her Old Woman self in and out of wherever she wanted to go and be and leave. Yehauweh traveled to Medicine Wheel gatherings where people fawned over her beadwork. Women's music festivals were her favorite! The crafts, the songs, the family—of women! The energy of contemporary woman-centered culture—ahhh, so close to, yet different from, her own origins. She breathed it all in. And she exhaled—her whole self! There she didn't hesitate a second when invited to strip her girdle-less body of its woman-painted clothing and waltz her soft round naked self among the young and younger. "This is what it's really about, Girls, being so comfortable in your skin no matter how it's hanging!"

And the Sister Circles of the Star Sisterhood—those were sacred. "But then," she would quip, "everything's sacred!" as she squatted to pee by her car in the parking lot of the retreat center her Daughter had reserved for a private Star-Sister Thanksgiving. (The mortified look on her Daughter's face was payment in full for all the "world's longest menopause" remarks made during. . .the world's longest menopause.) "Honey, just wait until you get to be where I am now. And bring a tissue, or a leaf, or something, because you'll probably have to pee."

It was a Good Old Age. And she was enjoying being good at it.

More often than not, she began to truly need help carrying her bags and walking up a hill or down. And that was okeh too. She had a circle of Helpers well trained by then. And her Helpers loved helping her.

Her own Mother had long since traveled the Starry Road to the Spirit World. She'd even left a sympathy card in the safe deposit box, informing her Daughter that it's okeh to grieve, then get over it—because "I'll be seeing you again soon enough. Enjoy your time here while you have it. . ." She returned every so often to help out, such as the time she woke up the Grand-Daughter when the house next door was on fire and flames were spitting onto the roof of what had been her own home. She had probably been close by anyway, as it was her birthday, and Spirits like to circle back around the holidays, to share in the festivities and see if anybody remembers them.

Yehauweh's Daughter was moving along her own Medicine Path, choosing animals as her patients or rather having them choose her. Yehauweh insisted her Daughter, Sister, Friend also become her Medicine Woman during her parade of illnesses and recoveries. (Tending puking buzzards proved to be easier, as the ego-tango of Mother and Daughter took no pause even in the emergency room. But the Bond endured. The Love.)

The time came for Yehauweh to move on to the next life. That day Yehauweh asked her Daughter if she thought she was dying now. And next she asked if her Daughter was ready to let her go. She felt fine. Had enjoyed her birthday party. But her heart was growing tired…so tired…too tired. A Spirit then entered the room and told Yehauweh it was soon time to go and that her Daughter would be okeh.

Like so many celebrations in her life, of her life, Yehauweh enjoyed being bathed by hands that loved her. Smiled as her hair was brushed with smell 'ums. Blushed as she was told she was beautiful. Laughed at her Daughter's family jokes. Took in all the bountiful "birthday" gifts that surrounded her. Minutes later, in the last exhale that matched her life's first inhale, Yehauweh gave it all back, left it all behind, stepped through the next doorway, with the confidence and grace only a Good Old Woman can carry. There were no pauses, no clinging to what was, no fear of what would become. There was only a starry path lit by the Love that she carried with her, the Love that met her, and the Love she left behind—as Love, she had become.

Yehauweh's Daughter held the fresh ashes of her Mother in her lap. The blood of her own body began to soak through her garments. She had never had the woes other women had spoken of—never had cramps, "PMS," or any discomfort since she began her moon-time at age nine. But then, she'd been raised in a Moonlodge Society and made friends early with the Spirits and herbs that ensured her well-being. And now she was flowing, gushing, bleeding heavily. She soaked through towels, one every twenty minutes. Was her body, in its grief over the moving-on of her Mother, giving up all its own dreams of children, all at once? Or was she being called to move into Elderhood—a crash course—as there were now no Elders left in her lineage? She had to become her own.

Whatever the reasons, she would later note that she had had "the world's shortest menopause on record—three days." No hot flashes, no mood swings, other than the expected grieving over the passage of her Mother, no "symptoms" other than a total emptying of her womb's sacred slurry. Had her lifelong herbal and nutritional care supported/prompted this swift passage? And/or had her Mother's fast passing co-created an energy shift that also propelled this deep, fast, thorough transition in her own life? She surmised that like all else in life, there were more than three reasons for anything. She was content with one or two, and the knowledge that life is a great mystery that need not be "solved" anymore than menstruation, menopause, and all the other experiences of womanhood need to be "cured." Respect and Honor had been her lineage's preferred responses to the mysteries and the knowledge, the questions and the answers of life on this female planet, the Mother Earth. That was good enough for her.

And still is.

I am Yehauweh's Daughter.

And I share her with You, not as a "Nyah-nyah-nyah-nyah—look at the matriarchy I inherited!" but as a gift from that matriarchy to You who walk this land, drink of her waters, are sustained by her vibrant foods and sweet air and sustaining gravity and lunar cycles and untamed love for *You*. Of the thousands and thousands of women I have met on my Medicine Journey, I have yet to meet more than a handful of women who have had their own natural life passages honored and celebrated by their own family. They have discovered their moon-times without the honoring of others, and carried them for decades as personal burdens, shame, pain, inconvenience, or embarrassment. They have never heard their own sweet name chanted by an Elder as she sings for their protection. And today, by the millions, they are again bravely walking into the uncharted territory of their lives, "menopause," without the honoring they, the honoring *You*, are due—honoring by your family, your friends and colleagues, your society and government, your health-care providers, and—your self.

It must be difficult to instantly create meaningful ritual of honoring for yourself. Not impossible, but lopsided if you have not first been so honored at some earlier point in your lives. And that is why I give Yehauweh's story to you, for you.

If I could, I would take you back to that time when you were a Little-Girl-Becoming-Woman, and I would sing for you, surprise you with gifts, wrap you in a fine soft robe, take you to the forest at night and introduce you to all your waiting Aunties. They would bless you with the treasures they hold in trust for you and all women. And we would feast and laugh and dance and cry and all the Old Ones who have already walked where you were headed would be there for you, their eyes twinkling like fireflies lighting the path ahead. And so, when you got to that place on your path where your next steps take you to your White-hair Wisdom, you would have the echo of all the Old Ones who have loved you, guided you, and are now beckoning you forward again. I would do that, and so much more for You—because you are a Woman on a female planet, the Mother Earth, and you deserve nothing less than Honor, Respect, Acceptance, Protection, Encouragement, and a Supportive Circle to witness your own self re-creation.

May you reread Yehauweh's story as your own. And where you find you ache for some aspect of it—the approval, the love, the gifts and attention, the belonging, an Elder chanting your name to the Moon, the innate respect and honor, the acceptance of all that you are, whatever yearnings emerge—may you find the Spirits of the Old Ones rising from these pages and encircling you with all that you need. Their love and wisdom transcend the human mind's notion of time and space. They are as close to you now as you allow them to be. And they already know your name: "Beloved Daughter, Sacred Woman."

AmyLee continues to honor the tradition of her Grandmothers through various offerings including:

www.HerNativeRoots.com
An interactive, educational health and healing website featuring her product line of certified organic and ethically wildcrafted herbals—Her Native Roots. Includes Herbs for Women—ensuring comfort in every phase of life!

www.SongPods.com
AmyLee has created "SongPods," musical and spiritual instruments that combine sacred sound with treasures from Mother Earth's sacred places.

www.MedWom.com
The webcast has archives from some of AmyLee's sharings, and a calendar of upcoming events and offerings.

www.SisterhoodoftheShields.net
A taste of spiritual legacy and an invitation to feast!

CHAPTER THREE

HORMONAL CYCLES: ROOTED in the WHEEL of LIFE

OUR LIVES ARE A PROGRESSION OF CIRCLES, EACH ELEGANTLY CYCLING within the others. Hormones link us with the "small" circle of life, our personal life journey. We pass from childhood into the moon-driven cycles of adolescence and adulthood. As hormones fluctuate again, we transition into "moon-pause," the changing woman years when we are more than adult and not yet elders. Finally we move into elder years, sinking deep taproots to nourish the coming generations. Ancient cultures recognized the power of these hormonal transitions and described them as "blood mysteries." This small circle roots us in present time.

The next circle, or "wheel," links us with our ancestors. Our ancestral lineage roots us in the past and prepares us for the future. We stand upon the foundation of our elders. They are the stones and fertile soil that give us ballast and nourishment.

The next largest wheel encompasses our relationship with the earth and the macrocycles of life. This larger wheel of planetary life informs both the personal and ancestral cycles we will explore later in this chapter.

Spirit, God, Goddess, All That Is, whatever you name the largest wheel of life, spins around and within all of the other cycles. This ever-present force encompasses and informs all aspects of creation as well as the past, present, and future. I hope you will catch whispers of this whirling force in each section of this book—in the "scientific" as well as the "spiritual" information, and in the individual women's words. We will discuss the third and fourth wheels of life in more depth in chapter 4.

HORMONES AND THE "SMALL" CIRCLE OF LIFE

Hormonal changes dramatically impact the body, influencing mood, energy, and mental clarity. Anyone who has witnessed a child's passage into her adolescent years (or remembers her own) can attest to the life-altering power of hormones. In contrast to a teenager's skyrocketing hormones, some women transitioning through perimenopause into menopause experience the dramatic effects of declining hormones.

Before discussing how hormones communicate, let's briefly define the terms menopause, perimenopause, and reproductive age. We will explore these stages in more detail in chapter 7.

- **Menopause**: One year with no menstrual bleeding. In this culture, the average age for menopause is fifty-one years old.

- **Perimenopause**: Literally "around the time of menopause." This is a transitional phase that can last from six months to ten years. A woman still has menstrual cycles, but the length of the cycle and many other factors may be changing.

- **Reproductive years**: Age during which women ovulate, bleed regularly, and have the potential to become pregnant.

Each hormone delivers a particular set of messages, affecting specific cells in different ways. Hormones bind to receptor sites, located on the outer surface of cell walls. The receptors are specifically "coded" or shaped to receive certain molecules. Progesterone receptors, for example, are shaped to receive progesterone molecules. No other hormone will bind at that receptor site. A hormone binding with a receptor is a bit like a key inserted into a lock; it opens the door to catalyze specific activities in the cell. Another way of visualizing receptors is as baseball mitts that project from the cell surface, waiting for the perfect "ball" (specific hormone) to catch.

With a clear understanding of how hormones function, you can begin to predict how the body will change when hormone levels fluctuate. We will now discuss the effects of four hormones produced by the ovaries (estrogens, progesterone, testosterone and inhibin) and two produced by the pituitary gland (follicle-stimulating hormone and leutenizing hormone).

Estrogens

What's the first hormone you think about when you hear the words "women's health"? Almost invariably the answer is "estrogen." The medical darlings of the past four decades, estrogens have numerous effects in the body.

SOURCES OF ESTROGENS AND ESTROGENIC ACTIVITY

- Ovaries

- Adrenal glands

- Skin

- Fat cells

- Xenoestrogens (includes estrogens in animal products)

- Prescription drugs (hormone replacement therapy [HRT], birth control pills)

Estrogens are a class of compounds that bind to estrogen-receptor sites. During reproductive years, the ovaries produce most of the estrogen in your body. The adrenal glands, skin, and other tissues make a small backup supply. Fat cells convert androstenedione, another steroid hormone, into estrogen. You can also absorb some estrogen in your diet, such as from meat products, particularly beef and chicken injected with estrogens before slaughter. Supplemental estrogens must be prescribed; estrogens are not available over the counter.

Your body produces three major estrogens: estrone, estradiol, and estriol.

- E_1 Estrone: The second strongest of the major estrogens, estrone is the most potentially carcinogenic. After menopause, estrone levels disproportionately increase compared to the other two estrogens as the adrenal glands take over more estrogen production.

- E_2 Estradiol: The strongest of the three estrogens, estradiol has the most effect on maintaining bone-mineral density. When taken orally, estradiol breaks down into estrone in the small intestine. Estradiol also converts to estrone (estrone-3-glucuronide) when broken down in the liver.

- E_3 Estriol: The weakest of the three estrogens, estriol has about 40 percent (less than half) the strength of estradiol. When taken by mouth, estriol does not convert to estrone in the small intestine but rather absorbs across the intestine wall intact. Estriol may protect against breast and endometrial cancer by competing with the stronger estrogens for receptor sites.

ESTROGENS' MESSAGES

In general, estrogens stimulate tissues to build, grow, and multiply. Outlined below are estrogens' effects on several major organs and systems in the body:

- **Uterus**: Estrogens stimulate the uterus and endometrium (lining of the uterus) to grow.

- **Breast**: Estrogens signal breast cells to "Divide, divide, divide. Don't bother fully developing, just keep dividing." Keep in mind that a cancer cell is an extremely rapidly dividing, extremely poorly developed cell. Women who take estradiol or estrone alone ("unopposed estrogen") for a long period of time increase their risk of developing breast cancer. Their breast cells receive only one message, "Divide, divide, divide," which starts edging those cells in the direction of breast cancer. Taking unopposed estrogen does NOT, however, guarantee a woman will develop breast cancer. After three years on estrogen replacement therapy (ERT), however, her risk for developing breast cancer significantly increases. She remains at greater risk for ten to fifteen years after stopping ERT.[1, 2]

- **Endocrine**: Estrogens increase blood-sugar levels. If blood-sugar levels remain elevated for a period of time, the body synthesizes fats—triglycerides and cholesterol—with the excess blood glucose.

- **Fat distribution**: Estrogens tell the body to deposit fat, particularly in the breasts and hips.

- **Sodium metabolism**: Estrogens signal the body to hold onto sodium, which in turn causes water retention. Excessive estrogen activity leads to bloating and edema.

- **Bone**: Our bones are constantly being broken down and rebuilt, broken down and rebuilt. The bones are like houses that are partly demolished and partly reconstructed every day. Osteoclasts (the "demolition crew") are cells that break down bone mineral to deliver calcium to the blood stream, while osteoblasts (the "construction crew") rebuild bone mineral. The problem as you grow older is that the demolition work starts outrunning the rebuilding crew, i.e. you lose more bone than you replace. Estrogens' job is to block osteoclasts, the demolition crew. Because estrogens blocks bone demolition, estrogens help maintain bone mineral density. Contrary to popular belief, estrogens do not help build bone mineral.

♦ **Nervous system**: In the central nervous system, estrogens have a "neuroexcitatory" effect. Estrogens stimulate and excite nervous-system activity. In excessive amounts, estrogens go beyond stimulating to irritating the central nervous system, causing anxiety, irritability, and nervousness.

ESTROGENS AND MENOPAUSE

By the onset of menopause (one year with no menstrual bleeding), estrogen levels have dropped 40 to 60 percent.

Progesterone

Progesterone has many opposite, balancing effects to estrogens. Progesterone also sends many messages that have nothing to do with estrogens, messages that are unique to progesterone.

SOURCES OF PROGESTERONE

♦ Ovaries

♦ Adrenal glands

♦ Myelin sheath

♦ Supplementation (over-the-counter and prescription)

During reproductive years, the ovaries produce most of your progesterone. The adrenal glands make a small backup supply. Unlike estrogens, progesterone is available over the counter in amounts that mimic the body's usual production ("physiological amounts," equal to what the body normally, naturally produces). Pharmacological amounts, that is, beyond what the body normally produces, require a prescription.

PROGESTERONE'S MESSAGES:

♦ **Uterus**: Progesterone has three effects on the lining of the uterus. When progesterone levels are high, the message for the endometrium is to slow down and hold on. The drop in progesterone levels at the end of the menstrual cycle signals the lining to shed completely.

♦ **Breast**: For breast cells, progesterone's message is "Slo-o-o-w down. Fully develop." Supplementing progesterone with estrogens slows breast-cell proliferation[3] and reduces breast cancer rates.[4] Low progesterone levels in reproductive-aged women are linked with a fivefold increase in pre-menopausal breast cancer.[5] Synthetic progestins, however, increase breast-cancer rates.[6,7] (In chapter 4, we will discuss the difference between progesterone and synthetic progestins). The conventional medical wisdom of prescribing estrogens alone for a woman after a hysterectomy makes little sense if she still has breasts.

◆ **Endocrine**: Progesterone stabilizes blood-sugar levels and encourages the body to use stored fat for energy.

◆ **Sodium metabolism**: Progesterone normalizes sodium levels and therefore stabilizes water metabolism.

◆ **Nervous system**: In the central nervous system, progesterone has a calming effect. In excessive amounts, progesterone goes beyond calming to sedating, causing sleepiness or lethargy. Research in France demonstrates that the myelin sheath produces a small but important amount of progesterone.[8,9] The myelin sheath protects nerve cells, acting like insulation around electrical wires. Studies show that nerve cells regenerate more quickly with supplementation of progesterone and anti-inflammatory medications. This combination speeds nerve-cell regeneration more effectively than either one by itself.

◆ **Libido**: Sexual desire increases when progesterone levels rise.

◆ **Thyroid**: Progesterone encourages the body to use thyroid hormone more efficiently.

Progesterone does not cause an increase in thyroid production, but rather makes the thyroid hormone receptors more sensitive so they better utilize the available thyroid hormone.

PROGESTERONE AND MENOPAUSE
Even before menopause, progesterone levels drop to almost nothing.

Testosterone
Men and women both produce estrogen, progesterone, and testosterone. The difference between us is the amount of the three hormones we produce, which in turn determines how we develop.

SOURCES OF TESTOSTERONE

♦ Ovaries

♦ Adrenal glands

♦ Skin

♦ Liver

The ovaries produce the majority of testosterone in a woman's body. The adrenal glands produce some testosterone, and the liver, skin, and other tissues synthesize small amounts.

FUNCTIONS OF TESTOSTERONE

♦ **Ovaries**: Studies have demonstrated that testosterone blocks the overgrowth of tumor cells in the ovary, thereby reducing the risk of developing ovarian cancer. If testosterone and other androgens do indeed suppress carcinoma, the development of ovarian cancer may be related to the ovaries' failure to produce enough androgens (for example, testosterone) after menopause.[10]

♦ **Hair**: Testosterone encourages both facial and body-hair growth.

♦ **Voice**: Testosterone deepens the voice.

♦ **Endocrine**: Testosterone encourages the body to store fat in the waist area.

♦ **Bone**: Like progesterone, testosterone stimulates osteoblasts, the "construction crew" in the bone. For men, decreased testosterone levels have been linked with osteoporosis[11], and recent research has explored the role of testosterone in increasing bone-mineral density in women. Researchers concluded that the combination of estradiol and testosterone would increase bone-mineral density, even after years of oral estrogen replacement therapy.[12] (Remember that estrogens maintain but do not build bone-mineral density.)

♦ **Libido**: Progesterone and testosterone also share the function of increasing libido, or sexual desire.

TESTOSTERONE AND MENOPAUSE

As you transition through perimenopause and into menopause, the part of the ovary that produces estrogen and progesterone begins to shut down, while the section of the ovary that makes testosterone remains relatively unaffected. In fact, the ovaries produce about 15 percent more testosterone after menopause. Because testosterone levels remain fairly constant while estrogen and progesterone levels drop, perimenopausal women have a relative increase in testosterone levels. You are not pumping out significantly more testosterone; instead, you may experience a relative increase in testosterone activity as estrogen and progesterone levels drop, "unmasking" testosterone-like effects in your body.

Leutenizing Hormone (LH)

The pituitary gland produces leutenizing hormone, which stimulates the ovarian follicle (a tiny, balloonlike structure on the ovary's surface) to burst and release an egg at the time of ovulation. LH then catalyzes the transformation of the follicle into the corpus luteum, which begins to produce progesterone. We will explore leutenizing hormone's activity in more depth in chapter 4.

Follicle-Stimulating Hormone (FSH)

Made by the pituitary gland, follicle-stimulating hormone also encourages the follicle to burst at the time of ovulation. FSH catalyzes the transformation of the ruptured follicle into the corpus leuteum, which then begins to produce progesterone.

Estrogen and FSH have an inverse relationship. When estrogen levels drop, FSH levels rise, catalyzing estrogen production in the ovaries. High estrogen levels trigger a negative feedback loop to decrease FSH production. In late perimenopause, FSH levels may soar, causing an increase in estrogen production. Jerilyn Prior, MD, hypothesizes that

> the perimenopausal ovary, instead of shriveling, goes through a grand finale. Although described as a "finale," the ovary continues to be a productive endocrine organ for many years. It makes estrogen, testosterone and weaker androgens well into old age. The perimenopausal ovary produces erratic and excess levels of estrogen, with unpredictable moods, heavy flow, hot flashes and mucous

symptoms that appear suddenly and unexpectedly. It seems that the remaining ovarian follicles are flogged into hormonal production by rising (but inconsistent) levels of follicle-stimulating hormone (FSH) produced in the pituitary gland.13

INHIBIN AND FSH

During reproductive years, the ovary produces inhibin, a hormone that moderates FSH levels. In late perimenopause, inhibin production decreases. As a result, FSH levels skyrocket, and estrogen production in the ovary soars. Combined with the drop in progesterone production, the increase in estrogen synthesis may exacerbate "estrogen dominance" symptoms, which we will explore in more detail chapter 7.

Increased FSH levels may be one of many causes of perimenopausal hot flashes. A surge of FSH causes a spike in estrogen production. Hot flashes may occur when estrogen levels plummet back to normal after the unusually high estrogen peak stimulated by the FSH surge. We know, however, that FSH is not the only trigger for hot flashes because they may continue even after FSH levels have returned to normal.

FEMALE REPRODUCTIVE HORMONES CHART

As we have learned, hormones affect different regions of the body in different ways. To review the functions of the three main female reproductive hormones, please refer to the chart below.

ANCESTORS, THE SECOND WHEEL OF LIFE

Much of this chapter has explored the "mechanics" of the body's hormonal transitions. A deeper aspect of the journey is exploring how these cycles spiral through the generations encoded in our DNA, the second, "ancestral," wheel of life. Hormonal transitions can link us with the larger ancestral cycles that shaped our origins and govern our evolution. Our biology influences the navigation of our destiny.

Menopause is one of many life "gates" we pass through. For women, our physical bodies deeply influence these life transitions. Men also go through similar passages, but their body changes are not as dramatic.

FUNCTIONS OF FEMALE REPRODUCTIVE HORMONES

	ESTROGEN	PROGESTERONE	TESTOSTERONE
UTERUS	Builds lining	Decreases build up of lining Encourages lining to shed fully (non-pregnant uterus) Maintains lining of uterus (pregnancy; prevents break through bleeding)	
BREASTS	Increases rate of cell division Decreases cell differentiation (maturation)	Decreases rate of cell division Increases cell differentiation (maturation)	
ENDOCRINE	Increases blood sugar levels	Decreases blood sugar levels	
FLUIDS	Increases sodium and water retention	regulates water metabolism	
BONE	Blocks activity of osteoclasts (cells that break down bone to deliver calcium to the blood stream)	Stimulates osteoblast activity, cells that lay down new bone	Stimulates osteoblasts (cells that lay down new bone)
CENTRAL NERVOUS SYSTEM	Physiological amounts cause "neuroexcitatory effect"; Pharmacological amount may cause irritability, mood swings	Physiological amounts have a calming effect Pharmacological amounts may cause sleepiness, lethargy, depression Increases libido (according to female mammal studies)	Increases libido and aggression
FAT DISTRIBUTION	Increases fat deposition in breasts, hips, buttocks		Increases fat deposition in waist and abdomen
VAGINA	Increases vaginal wall thickness and lubrication	Increases vaginal wall thickness and lubrication	

Blood Mysteries, Gateways of Life

Blood profoundly, visibly marks women's life transitions. Ancient peoples were awed that women could bleed and survive. What mysterious power allowed women to shed menstrual blood without dying? And what allowed them to retain that blood and transform it into a new child? Later in life, when menstruation ceased, the elder women could "hold their blood" to nourish wisdom that benefited the entire community.

Women hold the mystery of life right in their bellies. Life is not theoretical; life is *visceral.* Hormones guide and inform the blood mysteries. We have our own biology as a touchstone to track the rhythms and cycles of life.

Each gateway we pass through in our life journey holds the potential for wisdom and transformation. Obviously menopause, or moon-pause, the cessation of our moon-driven cycles, is not the only passage that offers the opportunity for transformation. For some women, puberty deeply changes them. For others, pregnancy and birth "cracks them open" in unexpected ways. Menopause is another passage that can deepen and expand our bodies, lives, and souls.

Some women experience transformation at other stages of their lives, too, completely unrelated to hormonal shifts. Kathleen Luiten (p. XXX) describes how a series of near-death experiences in her early twenties required her to develop body wisdom in order to survive. In comparison, other transitions were relatively calm passages in her life.

Approached with expectant awareness, each of the life gates we pass through can bless us with wisdom, grace, and power. If we go crashing through the gate, we may miss the subtle (and sometimes profound) gifts framing the doorway of the life passage.

Lizzy, a friend and beloved elder, surprised me one night when we were having dinner.

"I want to be a good root," she commented.

"What do you mean, Lizzy?" I asked.

"I want to be a good root for my children and grandchildren. I want them to have strong stock to grow from. I want to be a good root in our family tree."

I was delighted at how she relished this position, becoming a grounded source of inspiration, history, and strength for her family. I realized that in this menopausal transition, I would begin the evolution from branch to root in my own family tree.

I am blessed to stem from a lineage of strong, able women. My great-grandmother was an herbalist who kept a black bag by the door, ready to mount her horse night or day to assist at a birth or death, or to "doctor" a gravely ill neighbor. According to family lore, a great-great-aunt on my father's side sneaked into classes at the University of Michigan School of Medicine in the late 1800s, before women were officially admitted. She sat under desks at the back of the lecture halls and took notes. When she passed all of the medical exams, the university could not deny her a degree. She practiced as an ophthalmologist in Toledo, Ohio, and became a well-known philanthropist. When she developed a formula for a prescription eye drop, family members urged her to patent it, but she refused, as she wanted to make the formula available to as many people as possible.

Many of our family have been single, singular women, long before that stance was accepted or fashionable. Each generation has spawned at least one unmarried, or briefly married, woman. I'm that lone duck in the current generation. My great-great-aunt Annie lived and worked as a single woman in Columbus, Ohio in the late nineteenth century. After being diagnosed with breast cancer, Annie came home to live with her sister Clara, who was a childless farmwife.

"I feel they had a little sunshine in two dreary lives," wrote my great-aunt Eleanor, their niece, "a time when together they banished the loneliness of a spinster and a childless farm woman. What 'icebergs' live below such 'uneventful' lives!"

Clara continued to set a place for her sister at the dinner table years after Annie had passed.

My great-aunt Loey (Lois) never married. She worked as director of several nonprofits, then went home to help her parents in their later years. She became second mother to my mother and her siblings. In her eightieth year, she was honored (belatedly) by her alma mater, Ohio Weslyan, for serving as the captain of three teams during her college years: softball, basketball, and field hockey.

On the night my great-aunt Loey died (and before I knew that she had passed), I dreamed that three generations of sisters in my family were traveling together. Aunt Loey and her sister Gladys (my grandmother); my mother and her sister, Muffy; and my sister, Ruth, and I were all driving together in a 1950s sedan. We stopped at a roadside inn for the night.

While the others unpacked, I wandered outside in the late summer evening, enjoying the golden light as it slanted across the meadow behind the inn.

I found a claw-foot bathtub at the back of the property and was delighted to discover that the hot-water tap worked. I undressed, dropping my clothes in the grass, and stepped into the steaming tub. As I was soaking in the tub, one of the maids working at the inn stopped to chat.

"You're tourists, aren't you?" she asked, smiling. "You and the other women?"

I looked up at her. "No," I answered decisively. "We are travelers with a purpose."

The clarity of the dream has stayed with me for years. Each of those women, most of whom have now passed into spirit, focused her life on service. I knew from that moment on we were bonded by more than biology: we had a common devotion to serving and bettering the world.

Discover the roots in your own family. If you are blessed to have living elders, make time to visit them and record their memories. I wish now that I had spent more time with my grandmother in her last years, before Alzheimer's spirited her keen mind away. I treasure her stories about the Ohio farm where she grew up; the horse she rode to a neighboring town for Shakespeare and elocution lessons; and the building of Highway 40, the first road to connect the East Coast with the "new west."

Take a tape player, old family photos, and some fine tea when you visit the "roots" in your family. The depth and richness of these women's stories may surprise you. This is good practice for becoming a root yourself.

Have "The Talk" with Your Mother

When I began teaching nationally about perimenopause, menopause, and bio-identical hormones, my mother made a point of sharing her own experience.

"I had a *really* hard time," she commented. "You probably don't remember that period, but I was really depressed. I was in my mid-forties, and I had absolutely no energy. Because I had had a hysterectomy, the doctor didn't think about menopause. I didn't have periods to signal that my hormones were changing. He ordered the Glycola test for hypoglycemia, which just about did me in. I realized later that I was allergic to the corn syrup and cola in the drink. Then he ordered the menopause test (FSH) and realized I was moving into menopause. It was an awful time, and my mother had never said anything to prepare me for it."

"Maybe Grandma didn't have a hard time," I said.

My mom closed her eyes and creased her brow, as if trying to ward off a bad dream. "Well, maybe she didn't. I just know it was a really difficult time."

Having "the talk" with your mother about her experience of menopause may be healing for both of you. My mother transitioned through menopause when few women even whispered the words "the Change." Certainly my mother never discussed menopause with her own mother. I'm still not certain whether my grandmother's silence was out of social grace or lack of noteworthy comment.

Remember that your mother's experience of menopause does *not* predict your own. We inherit the biological *timing*. We will go into menopause around the same age our mothers, grandmothers, and great-grandmothers went into menopause. The quality of the transition, though, can vary radically. Just because my mother had an "awful" experience of menopause does not mean that I will. Her age at the time of menopause, though, will predict my own timing.

Living History

I offer the following guidelines for reflecting on your own life journey up to this point. I also encourage you to contact relations—your mother, grandmothers, aunts, cousins—to ask for their stories. You are weaving herstory, recording the ancestral passage that continues through your own blood and ovaries.

Remember that all of the eggs in your ovaries developed by the time you were a three-month-old fetus. Your own children's health was influenced while you were in utero. If you carry a daughter in your womb, your grandchildren's health and vitality is affected before your daughter is ever born. Your ancestors' evolution continues through your own body.

MARK YOUR REFLECTIONS

Take time to remember and reflect on the significant transitions in your life. Write your reflections in your journal or a notebook. Or, if writing is not your primary form of expression, consider drawing, painting, or making music that expresses your experience of these important life transitions.

◆ Reflect on your first menstrual period. Do you remember where you were when you first discovered blood in your underpants or on the toilet paper? Do you remember the days or weeks leading up to that time? Who did you tell? How did they react? What messages did you receive about your body and your bleeding? Did your friends and family celebrate your first blood with you?

◆ Reflect on when you became an "adult." For some, this may be graduation from a school; for others, it may a first job. Travel, relationships, financial changes (for example, buying a house) may also signal your passage into adult years.

◆ Did you become a mother? Your creation may have been a human child or the birthing of a career. Even without conception or delivery, you may have been mother to many. Did you conceive and then lose a child? What does mothering, nurturing, and creating mean for you? How did your menstrual cycles influence this part of your life? Were you plagued with cramps or other menstrual problems? Were you able to tap into the fecund, creative power of your bleeding time?

◆ If you are still bleeding, how do you relate to your cycles now? How have your rhythms changed since you began bleeding as a young woman?

◆ Ask your relatives about their own passages:

◆ **Menarche/Moon Time**: Do they remember when they started bleeding? What were they told about their bodies, their blood? Did they have a ritual to mark the first moon-time?

◆ **Mother/Adult**: When did they become adults? Did they choose to be mothers? Would they do anything differently if they had their lives to live over? Did they struggle with societal expectations or move happily with them? Would they make different choices if they were young adults now, in this day and age?

◆ **Menopause/Moon-pause**: What was their menopausal passage like? What do they wish they had been told, or wish they had been able to say during that time? What wisdom do they have to offer you now, at this stage in *your* life passage?

♦ You may choose to make a special book or series of letters for your own daughters (and sons, too) to share your life wisdom. You could put these letters away to be opened on specific days, for example, your daughter's first moon-time, the day she discovers she is pregnant, or the moon-drenched night she gives birth to a child. You could write letters for your son to open the first day he drives a car, has a wet dream, or graduates from high school. You may choose to gift your children with a handbound book when they move into their own home, marry, or conceive a child. Let your intuition guide you. Seed your wisdom for the generations to come, so that the ancestral soil they stand on will be rich with your offerings.

Reflections by Brooke Medicine Eagle

Brooke Medicine-Eagle is an American native earthkeeper, earth-wisdom teacher, visionary, sacred ecologist, songwriter, feng shui practitioner, and catalyst for wholeness, whose dedication is to bring forward the ancient truths concerning how to live a fully human life in sustaining harmony with All Our Relations. She is a member of Sacred Ground International, an educational foundation on her home Crow Reservation. The foundation supports energetic research as well as sustainable living and buffalo ranching. She is the author of a spiritual autobiography, Buffalo Woman Comes Singing. Her new book, The Last Ghost Dance, explores the transformational practices of earth magic and ascending into our greater humanity.

The primary, indigenous people's *culture*, rather than the "spiritual tradition," helped prepare me for menopause. Women from primary times honored the cycles of women's lives—birthing, maiden, mother, and crone. The culture clearly defined a woman's function in each cycle. This deep knowledge was as much about how to live and about how the society worked as it was about spirituality. Within this culture, though, were many spiritual components, including the receiving of spirit that was part of moon-time, our bleeding time. In the tape called "Moon Time," I have outlined a whole practice of the women's mysteries, about how to bring through wisdom when the veil is thin.

That background about working with our moon time, or bleeding time, is necessary to understand what I would express about menopause, or moon-pause. For the four or so days when a woman is on her moon-time, her function is to quiet herself, to go apart, to rest herself, to still herself from the outward world. The veil in her consciousness between All-That-Is and her daily life is the thinnest at the time when she is bleeding, at the dark of the moon. If she is being guided by the great cycles and the moon, then bleeding comes on the dark of the moon.

So a woman, bleeding at the dark of the moon, is the clearest channel and the closest to Creator, All-That-Is, the Great Spirit, the Great Knowledge, the Great Source, the Great Knowing that any human being ever is naturally.

The moon—time is not only a time for a woman to rest, to quiet herself, and to deepen her spirit, but it is also a time for her to act as a channel for information from Source. Women in their moon-time, in their bleeding time, are dreaming and calling vision. I'm asking now not only for myself, but for the people. Other times I can pray for myself, but in these four days I'm asking to be a hollow bone to let through, to birth through me the knowledge that's needed for my people.

This incredibly powerful experience is something that we are very much missing in this day and age. Four days out of the month, *every month*, the moon-time woman went deeply into spirit and meditation. It would be like completing thirteen vision quests a year.

During moon-pause, or menopause, the society freed you to connect with Source even more of the time. You no longer had a family to raise; you had less outward work to do. You left those more outward responsibilities behind and were given the opportunity to be more deeply with spirit. Certainly many of the grandmothers still did beautiful beading, offering a prayer with every bead, but the heavier outward responsibilities of caring for others was left behind. The moon-pause woman was the highest and finest visionary.

And each woman, as we all do, brought through insights related to her. If she was a pottery maker, then she might have an inspiration during her moon-time about how to make a pot more waterproof with pitch. Or a weaver might discover a better way of weaving. Another woman might receive a vision, a "head's up" about preparing for a change, or spiritual information.

In our time, I'm a very poor example of this slowing down and listening. In the world I was asked to inhabit, I've been flying across the world, carrying as much light as I can. I have not had a yin, quiet life at all. It's taken me a while to slow down as I've gone into my moon-pause.

Moon-pause was interesting to me because I'm very androgynous. One of the gifts I've been told I have, one of the primary gifts, is the balance of my energy form and the high spin that results from that balance. That high spin generates a kind of intensity that helps things change around it, just like a little tornado. Combining that energy with positive intention can move things in a really powerful way.

Perhaps that androgyny is part of why I always had very light periods. Some of my women friends whom I felt so sorry for would be sick with cramps and heavy bleeding. Oh, my gosh, it was such a challenging time for those gals. But I bled very little, just a brief time each month. Occasionally I would have some minor cramping, but it was not a difficult time for me. I was taken by surprise by my moon-pause time. I had one period that was like these gals I described. I mean I *bled*—down my legs. Then it stopped for two or three months. I think I had a couple regular periods or just a little spotting and then *poof,* that was it.

I didn't have much emotional experience, either, although at the time I knew enough to begin taking a very light, natural phytoestrogen. I laughed and said that my body had run so cold all my life that if I had hot flashes, I'd just think I was finally warming up. I had night sweats. That's one thing I really knew was different. I'd never had that happen before. But that was about the only thing I experienced.

What's been fascinating in my life is that I've stimulated a lot of moon circles and encouraged a lot of women to work with their moon-time and moon lodges, yet I haven't had a moon lodge myself because I've been on the road all my life. Around moon-pause, I did not have a specific group I wanted to have a ceremony with, so the transition into moon-pause hasn't been very ceremonial with me.

Last year I had an experience with a group of women at Sacred Ground, our home ranch on the Crow Reservation, where my girlfriend now lives. I have had a vision of becoming an earth-and-water dragon that brings in moisture, cares for the water, and nourishes life through moisture and water and rain. That image came, but I'd never been initiated with that vision. So the women took me up to this beautiful spring—it's one of the springs I remember from my childhood—and washed me, cleansed me, then painted me as a dragon. The ritual was very simple, and we really had a lot of fun doing it. But as we were doing it, we understood we were honoring this new cycle in my life, that is, my crone cycle.

My moon-pause transition has gone quite smoothly. Maybe it's because I haven't had children. As with many women in this culture, I've had a lot of experience, but I don't feel very wise or grandmotherly. I always tell people, "I'm your naughty aunt." I've never been a person whose predilection was nurturing, care taking, cooking, and all of that kind of thing.

The function of the grandmother lodge is also to pass wisdom to the young girls. The grandmothers are the ones who teach the granddaughters of the culture around their moon-time. I think somehow that's easier than working with your mom. The grandmother have amazing wisdom, and they bring the young along. Once again, I haven't been around a community with children. It's very interesting to think about how to touch in with the children and honor that part of the wise-woman function.

We almost have to express the moon lodge differently today just because of how we're living. It's challenging for women who are out in the world, on a schedule and having to work a job from 9 to 5, no matter what day it is. That schedule has really damaged our bodies, pressing and stressing them, and not taking time to rest. The function of the moon-time cannot be fulfilled because you can't sit somewhere for four days.

Can you imagine that? Four days with *nothing* to do. To be quiet and still, eat simple foods, drink lots of water, sit back and draw or vision, dream or nap. That kind of time is not available to many women in our modern times. And part of the challenge of honoring moon-time is that it requires a big community of support.

Among my people, the boys stay in the women's lodge until they are seven. The boys know how to cook and sew and do everything that needs to be done, at least in rudimentary form, by the time they are seven. So they are not dependent on someone else for those skills. Then they go into the men's lodge and continue to learn their primary skills. Grandmothers do not go into the moon lodge because they no longer have their moon-time. Younger girls are well trained in various things, as are the men and boys. No one has to take care of anyone else. So it takes the cooperation of a whole culture, a society, to afford women that time in the moon lodge.

The value of moon-time is not understood in the larger culture, in America and many other places. The feminine wisdom has not been valued. We've been in a time of masculine dominance. As I understand it in my own body and remembering, there was a time of feminine dominance, when the women kept the men as slaves to work hard, and studs for children. Then, of course, we've swung the opposite way, toward incredible masculine dominance. Now I'm told we are swinging back to balance, to more equality. It will be like the ancient matrilineal societies archeologist Marija Gimbutas found in eastern Europe where women seemed to be their leading shamans, yet everyone took part in everything. They were artists; they didn't have weapons. They just had beautiful skills, art, agriculture, and herbs. The skills seemed to be equally distributed between the men and women depending on what their heart and body wanted, not so much according to gender role.

We're coming back into a time of balance when the feminine wisdom will be honored again. It will be very powerful because some of the most amazing prophetic information came from women in their moon-time and from grandmother-lodge women who were visioning. Long ago women in their moon time saw cobwebs strung across the land; of course, that would be the power lines and telephone lines we have now. Women in their moon-time saw these and many other prophetic things, like silver birds in the sky that they didn't understand at all, that we would later know as airplanes.

I wish that I had had a grandmother lodge to see in action, to have a direct experience, rather than just being told about it. In my life, and in so many of my sisters' lives as well, there's a sadness that we didn't have those models to guide us from the time we were born.

This moon-pause transition is like going around the medicine wheel. For me, the east is dawning, illumination, morning light, bright ideas. Things come up from the darkness in the east. They're sprouts coming up from deep in the ground, children being birthed from their mother's belly. Everything is waking in the east.

The south, then, is warmth and summertime, midday, midsummer, growth, intense, relational, warm-hearted. The south is about activity, doing-ness. In the east you have an "aha," a bright idea, and in the south you put into action.

East and south are both yang. The east is the "little male," and the south is what I call the "big male," the really yang expression. No matter whether you are male or female, when you are really *doing,* you are in that yang mode.

Then you move into the little feminine, the west, where you begin to gather knowledge about what has happened. The west is evening, maturation, looking inward. West is the autumn, when we gather the harvest. Let's say you did a study on babies given breast milk or formula. In the west, you would gather the data. "Oh, twenty out of twenty-five did better on this milk." That would be gathering knowledge, seeing the facts.

Autumn looks within. First comes letting go, quieting, softening, like coming home from work in the late afternoon; then, you contemplate, reviewing the day and what you have learned or understood. You begin to see what you have gained at the level of knowledge, fact, and information. You are gathering the material harvest.

West is the beginning of the moon-pause work. But the really powerful moon-pause work is in the north, settling into quietness and allowing the knowledge to turn into wisdom. Knowledge is just individual facts, but wisdom is applying those facts in harmony with the whole of things, for the good of everything. You take the knowledge and put it to use.

So you might say, "Wow, healthy mothers who nurse their babies have healthier babies." Now, you could come up with many things based on that data, with the wisdom that, of course, that's the natural way. That is harmony. That's the way our bodies were made. The child comes close to the heart when it is put on the breast immediately after birth. That heartbeat is the baby's biological, emotional, and psychic connection. Its little head is laid there to hear that heart again, to connect it back to the heart it heard in the womb. Coming back again and again to that heartbeat sets up a deep connection, through the mother with the Earth and with the rest of life. That's a comforting, safe, nurturing, happy, restful place to stand in the world.

That wisdom, then, could be applied. "Aha! That gives me an idea." So, there you are again in the east, applying wisdom in the world.

The north is the grandmother-lodge function. Certainly we are gathering some of the information as we slow down from our working life, settling into the west. But really the grandmother lodge itself is in the north of the medicine wheel, transforming knowledge and experience into wisdom. Let it percolate deep in the stillness and the quietness. I think about sitting by White Buffalo Woman's fire, her wisdom lake, and deepening. That quiet stillness just naturally stirs the seeds and grows new understandings that can then be put into action. The grandmother probably wouldn't put them into action, but through her offering of those gifts and understandings to those younger than her, that wisdom can be used.

As you make the transition into moon-pause, tune in and be more connected with the moon, wherever you are. You could be flying in an airplane and watching the moon rather than working on your business. Just sit back on your flight and dream and vision; bring something through. It isn't ideal, but that's the kind of thing we can do. Awareness and knowledge make the difference. That's why I've tried to get out the information about women's mysteries, about moon time and moon-pause. Everyone, from medical doctors to native teachers, is bringing forward this information now, and a generation of women has had a chance to at least get a grasp on it.

Brooke can be contacted through her website www.bme.com or by regular mail: Brooke Medicine Eagle, 1 Second Avenue East, C401, Polson, MT 59860

CHAPTER FOUR

HORMONES: MESSENGERS of BIOLOGY, MESSAGES from SPIRIT

HORMONES ARE THE BODY'S MESSENGERS, DELIVERING CATALYTIC information to each cell of the body by stimulating changes in the cell without being changed themselves. In this chapter, we will explore how the hormones deliver messages and how best to supplement hormones (if needed). The hormones act as couriers without our conscious attention. Receiving messages from spirit, however, often requires conscious effort. The second part of this chapter focuses on how we can cultivate, like a patient gardener, our receptivity to the subtle whisperings of spirit.

HORMONES: THE BODY'S MESSENGERS

Your body produces two basic types of hormones: protein and fat-based hormones. Steroids, which include reproductive hormones, are fat-based hormones synthesized from cholesterol. Despite its current bad reputation, your body absolutely needs cholesterol for certain vital functions, including the production of steroid hormones. The adjacent chart shows the steroid hormones produced by the adrenal glands.

Look closely at the central part of each of the hormones. Note that the central structure of each molecule is exactly the same. Only the "tails" attached to the central molecule differ. These appendages "encode" the message a hormone delivers. Even a small change in this tail alters the message. Look, for example, at the difference between testosterone and estriol. What's the difference? Only the placement of **one hydrogen atom**. Changing the tail alters the message and therefore the hormone.

A simple way to visualize these steroid hormones is to imagine a Mr. Potato Head toy with a variety of pieces attached. Each piece is like a different "tail." If you change the piece (or "tail"), you change the message and therefore the hormone.

Hormones are messengers that deliver very specific signals throughout the body. They are the body's gossips, and each one has a different story to tell. The more of a particular hormone that is present, the louder its story is.

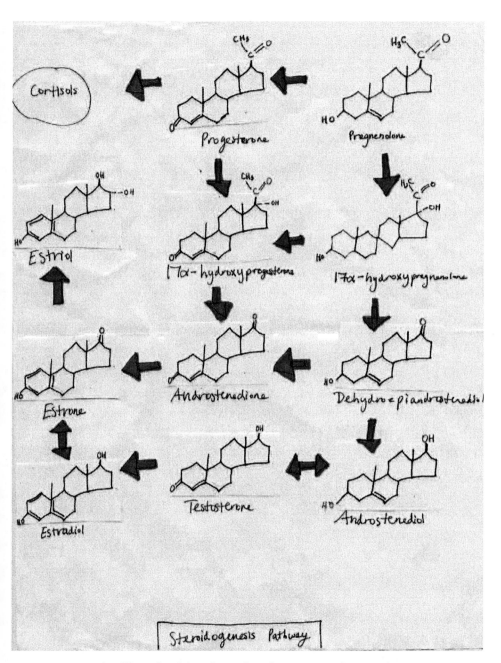

I will redo this chart for the second round

The lower the hormone level, the quieter that particular story is. All of the hormones are delivering messages at the same time. The relative amount of a particular hormone determines which story is loudest, and therefore which hormonal signal will predominate.

Natural vs. Bio-Identical Hormones

Thanks to recent media exposés, many women are asking their doctors for natural hormone prescriptions. Unfortunately the word "natural" is confusing. The health-food industry, much less the pharmaceutical industry, has never concisely defined the term.

Some insist that "natural" hormones are derived from plant sources. No plant, however, makes an exact duplicate of progesterone or testosterone. A few plants produce tiny amounts of the estrogens our bodies produce (for example, estrone in pomegranates), but certainly not enough to have a major therapeutic effect. We will discuss phytoestrogens, plant molecules that mimic but do not duplicate the estrogens we produce, in chapter 5.

A more useful term than natural is "bio-identical," meaning an exact duplicate of something made in our bodies. "Bio-identical" refers to hormones produced from any source that replicate the ones we make. Certain plant molecules can be altered in a laboratory to produce bio-identical hormones. Those same plants can also be used to synthesize molecules that do not exactly duplicate our endogenous hormones, for example, synthetic progestins. (See below for more information on progestins.) Using a plant base does not guarantee that the substance will be "natural" or, more precisely, "bio-identical."

The key issue for natural hormone replacement therapy is whether the hormone duplicates one made in our bodies. The source used to make the hormone is not as important as the final molecular structure.

What This Means for You

The source used to make a hormone is not as important as whether it is "bio-identical" (an exact duplicate of one of your body's hormones).

Progesterone, Synthetic Progestins, and Wild Yam

Unlike estrogens, which are a class of hormones, the body produces only one molecule of progesterone. Synthetic progestins, also known as progestogens, are similar enough to progesterone that they will bind at progesterone receptor sites. The progestins, however, have altered tails. Remember that changing a hormone's tail changes the message and therefore the function of the hormone. Of all of the messages progesterone delivers, progestins only know three:

◆ Slow the development of the endometrium (lining of the uterus). This is an important function, particularly at the time of menopause, because overgrowth of the endometrium increases the risk of developing uterine cancer.

◆ Stop the development of follicles in the ovary. Birth-control pills contain progestins to stop the development of the follicles and therefore ovulation.

◆ Stimulate osteoblast activity, which in turn increases bone-mineral density.

Other than these three messages, the progestins do not know all of the additional messages progesterone delivers, for example, stabilize blood-sugar levels, calm the central nervous system, or normalize water metabolism.

Progestins also do not slow the growth of breast tissue, so when combined with estrogens they do not decrease the risk of developing breast cancer. In fact, recent studies demonstrate that progestins actually increase the risk of breast cancer.[1,2]

Progestins, with their altered tails, also cause a whole range of additional side effects including edema, gallbladder congestion, nausea, fatigue, severe allergic reactions, increased facial hair, balding, hemorrhagic eruptions, and spasms of the coronary arteries.[3] Other side effects include an increase in PMS symptoms,[4] increased sodium retention,[5] and weight gain.

THE ECONOMICS OF PROGESTERONE AND PROGESTINS

Why do physicians prescribe progestins if these molecules deliver incomplete or altered messages? Unfortunately most physicians are not educated about the difference between synthetic progestins and progesterone. Many prescribe progestins and then are stymied when progesterone levels fail to rise. No matter how much progestin you take, progesterone will never rise *because progestins are not the same molecule as the progesterone your body makes.*

Pharmaceutical companies heavily influence conventional physicians' drug knowledge, and those companies are not particularly interested in

educating physicians about the difference between bio-identical progesterone and synthetic progestins. Unfortunately economics drives this
choice. If a pharmaceutical company makes an exact duplicate of one of
the hormones our bodies makes (and they do know how), they cannot
patent the molecule. Without a patent, the company cannot recoup their
research money. In contrast, the pharmaceutical companies can patent the
altered progestin molecules and therefore reap a great profit from their sale.
Each company "tweaks" the progestin's tail slightly differently so they can
patent their own particular progestin molecule.

PROGESTERONE AND WILD YAM

Early in the twentieth century, researchers tried unsuccessfully to extract
progesterone from animal placentas. The process was difficult and astro-
nomically expensive. During the Great Depression of the 1930s, progesterone cost $1000 a gram, if it was available. Because of scarcity and
expense, physicians rarely prescribed progesterone.

In the early 1930s, a research chemist named Dr. Russell Marker decided
to look for a plant source to synthesize progesterone. Aware that no plant
makes an exact duplicate of progesterone, Marker was seeking a plant that
had the correct central structure, the "Mr. Potato Head" common to all
steroid hormones. He literally searched around the world until he found the
Mexican wild yam species *Dioscorea*. From the wild-yam root, he extracted a
particular molecule called diosgenin (see chart, p. XXX). This molecule has
the right central structure, but notice the additional rings and tails stuck on
that central molecule. In a laboratory, Marker learned to alter the tails
attached to the diosgenin to make an exact duplicate of the progesterone
our bodies produce.

Marker's discovery was pure genius because our body does not know how
to convert wild yam into progesterone. We have our own synthetic pathways
for hormone production, and none of those pathways utilize diosgenin.

Eventually researchers learned to use diosgenin to make exact duplicates
of all the other steroid hormones by further altering the tails. Later
researchers discovered that certain molecules in soy also had the correct central molecule and could be used to synthesize bio-identical steroid hormones. Soy products in our diet, however, do not become estrogen or other
hormones in the body. The conversion from isolated soy molecule to bio-
identical hormone must happen in a laboratory.

A SHEEPISH COMPARISON BETWEEN
DIOSGENIN AND PROGESTERONE

Unfortunately certain supplement companies have circulated misleading information about the body's ability to convert certain herbs into steroid hormones. Wild yam and other herbs have wonderful botanical benefits, which we will discuss in more detail in chapter 5, but they do not magically transform into hormones in the body.

For those who are confused about the difference between wild yam and progesterone, consider the following analogy: taking wild yam and hoping it will become progesterone is like putting a sheep around your shoulders and hoping it will become a wool sweater. No matter how long you leave that sheep around your shoulders, it will not become a wool sweater. You can, however, take the sheep off your body, sheer the wool, card it, spin it, etc. and make a wool sweater. Similarly, in a laboratory the wild yam can be synthesized into a bio-identical molecule of progesterone. These alterations happen outside the body. The sheep will not change into a sweater on your shoulders, and the wild yam will not change into progesterone in your digestive system or skin, but each can be transformed outside the body.

If you are unsure whether a product contains wild yam or progesterone, carefully read the label. If it says "wild yam extract," you have the sheep, not the wool sweater. If the label lists "Progesterone," or "U.S.P. Progesterone," you have the sweater, the wild yam that has been converted in a laboratory to bio-identical progesterone. "U.S.P." simply means "United States Pharmacopoeia." The U.S. Pharmacopoeia catalogs all prescription and some over-the-counter medications. The Pharmacopoeia lists "U.S.P. Progesterone" and notes the molecular structure to differentiate bio-identical progesterone from the multitude of manufactured progestins.

PROGESTERONE AFTER A HYSTERECTOMY?

After a hysterectomy, most women receive a prescription for estrogen alone. Remember that many physicians confuse progestins and bio-identical progesterone. One of the few messages the progestin knows is to slow the development of the uterine lining. Obviously a woman after a hysterectomy has no uterine lining to worry about, so a progestin would be inappropriate.

My first concern, however, is whether the woman still has breasts. If she does, bio-identical progesterone would be very appropriate, particularly if she is taking estrogen replacement therapy. Estrogens' message for breast cells is "Divide, divide, divide. Don't bother fully developing, just keep dividing." In contrast, bio-identical progesterone tells breast cells to slow down and fully develop.[4] Progesterone decreases breast cancer rates in women receiving estrogen therapy.[5] As mentioned earlier, synthetic progestins may increase breast cancer risk.

Most definitely a woman may benefit from progesterone supplementation after a hysterectomy, particularly if she is taking estrogen. Like any perimenopausal or menopausal woman, she needs an individualized assessment of her symptoms and risk factors for osteoporosis to determine whether she needs any HRT.

The Scoop on Estrogen Prescriptions

In chapter 3, we discussed some of the major differences between estrone (E_1), estradiol (E_2) and estriol (E_3). In this chapter, we will explore different types of estrogen prescriptions and their effect on our bodies.

HORSE VERSUS HUMAN ESTROGEN

Only in the last forty years has Western medicine described menopause as a disease rather than a normal life passage. Unlike natural life transitions, "diseases" can be cured, and Premarin has been the late twentieth-century doctors' favorite menopause potion. Before the introduction of Viagra, Premarin was the most widely prescribed drug in the United States. Pharmacists continue to fill more prescriptions for Premarin than any cardiovascular, corticosteroid, or antibiotic drug.

Premarin is 17-hydroxy-equine (horse) estrogen (see diagram). "Pregnant mare's urine" becomes the word "Premarin." Wyeth Ayerst, the manufacturers of Premarin, keep pregnant mares in stalls and withhold water so that their urine is exceptionally strong, making the horse estrogen easier to extract.

Remember that altering a hormone's tail changes the message and therefore the hormone's effect. You can see that Premarin does not duplicate any of the three major estrogens (estradiol, estrone, or estriol) that our body produces. In addition, over half the estrogen in Premarin is an equine version of estrone, the most potentially carcinogenic of the three estrogens. Currently we have no studies comparing the effects of human and horse estrogen supplementation in human females. We do know the horse estrogens are more difficult for the human liver to break down and excrete.

Progestin

Progesterone

Diosgenin (isolated from wild yam)

Chemical Formula C₁₉H₂₂O₂

I will redo this chart for the second round

Although pharmaceutical companies cannot patent human estrogens, they are free to patent other animals' hormones, which has made Premarin a very lucrative prescription drug for Wyeth Ayerst.

PREMARIN ALTERNATIVES: TRI-EST

Jonathon Wright, MD, has championed a new approach to estrogen supplementation. He studied healthy women's urine and recorded the breakdown products (metabolites) of the three estrogens to determine their normal ratio. Keep in mind that urinary metabolites may or may not accurately reflect active hormone levels in the body. Through his research, Dr. Wright determined that the normal ratio of estrogen metabolites is 80 percent estriol, 10 percent estradiol and 10 percent estrone. He began prescribing this ratio of the three estrogens, which he named "Tri-est," for his patients who needed estrogen.[8]

No pharmaceutical manufacturers make Tri-est, but any compounding pharmacy can fill a physician's prescription for the three estrogens. Compounding pharmacies still make some of their own prescriptions, for example, special order creams, tablets, and suppositories. Check your local phone directory for information about compounding pharmacies.

ESTRIOL (E$_3$): PROTECTIVE AGAINST BREAST CANCER?

The weakest of the three estrogens, estriol, has about 40 percent of estradiol's strength. Estriol doses are usually three times higher than estradiol prescriptions to achieve similar effects.

The uterus secretes high levels of estriol during pregnancy, which may explain why women who have babies before age twenty-two have lower breast cancer rates. The estriol "set point" in these women presumably is higher than those who give birth later in life.[9] Because of its weaker hormonal signal, estriol may protect against breast and endometrial cancer by competing with the stronger estrogens for receptor sites.[10, 11]

In essence, estriol mimics the action of Tamoxifin, a drug prescribed for breast cancer (and now for breast-cancer prevention). Estriol, however, does not increase the risk of endometrial cancer, while Tamoxifin escalates endometrial cancer risk by seven and a half times (750 percent).[12]

In Europe and China, estriol is the preferred form of estrogen for hormone replacement therapy.

Forms of Hormone Supplementation

ORAL

Whether food, herb, or hormone, anything taken by mouth moves across the intestines into the bloodstream and then passes directly to the liver. One of the liver's many jobs is to break down and excrete hormones. Like everything else we ingest, the intestines absorb oral hormones and shunt them to the liver where most of the hormones are immediately broken down. The more hormones we ingest, the harder the liver has to work.

Steroid hormones, along with other fatty substances, exit the liver via bile. Increased bile production can in turn stress the gallbladder, the organ that concentrates and then discharges bile into the small intestine. Because of the increased workload, women taking oral hormones have an increased risk of developing gallstones or other gallbladder diseases.

Oral Estrogen Much of oral estradiol (E_2) converts to estrone (E_1), a weaker and more carcinogenic form of estrogen, in the small intestine. The liver then converts 35 to 95 percent of the estrogen into estrone-3-glucuronide. Oral estriol, the weakest of the three estrogens, passes across the intestinal mucosa intact.

Oral Progesterone When taken orally, progesterone crosses the intestinal wall and goes directly to the liver, where about 90 percent of the hormone is immediately broken down. Progesterone is exceptionally easy for the liver to break down, a fact that frustrated scientists trying to develop an effective form of oral progesterone for many years. Not until the 1980s did researchers develop a capsule of 200 mg of micronized (pulverized) progesterone suspended in vegetable oil that provided longer sustained levels of progesterone in the bloodstream.

Until recently, testing equipment could not differentiate between progesterone and its metabolites. Researchers are now discovering that sleepiness and lethargy, commonly associated with high progesterone levels, are more closely related to the amount of Iprogesterone metabolite than to progesterone itself. Because oral progesterone must be given in larger quantities, women taking oral progesterone are more likely to suffer from lethargy or depression than those taking the lower doses of transdermal progesterone.

TRANSDERMAL

Literally meaning "across the skin," this term refers to skin or vaginal application. Transdermal hormone applications also avoid the "first pass" through the liver and therefore can be prescribed in smaller amounts. Taking smaller doses reduces the workload for both liver and gallbladder.

Transdermal Estrogen As a comparison, an oral estrogen prescription must be at least twenty times higher than the Estraderm (estradiol) patch in order to be effective![13] Women with a history of uterine fibroids, however, should avoid estradiol patches, because increased estradiol levels may stimulate fibroid growth.[14] Oral estrogen supplements do not have the same effect, probably because a large portion of the estradiol is converted to estrone, a weaker form of estrogen, in the intestines. Some women are allergic to the adhesive on the patch. For those with skin sensitivities, a cream, gel, or vaginal suppository may be a more appropriate choice.

Transdermal Progesterone Applying progesterone through the skin or vaginal tissue avoids the first pass through the liver, allowing the hormone to travel through the body and bind with hormone receptor sites before being metabolized in the liver. The amount of transdermal progesterone needed to effect blood and saliva levels is much lower than oral progesterone. The average daily oral progesterone prescription is about five times more than the typical transdermal dose (200 mg oral vs. 40 mg transdermal).

Progesterone Vaginal Suppositories Blood levels of progesterone rise later and remain elevated longer with vaginal progesterone suppositories or cream compared with oral doses of progesterone. Progesterone levels in the blood remained in a narrower, more predictable range with vaginal administration.[15]

Gels Any of the steroid hormones can be prepared as a gel rather than a cream. Testosterone is most commonly prescribed in gel form.

SUBCUTANEOUS IMPLANT

This method involves surgically inserting a device under the skin that releases estradiol into the fatty tissue over a period of time. Researchers developed these implants for women who require higher plasma (blood) levels of estrogens. Estradiol levels rise rapidly, remain constant for about four months, and then decline.

If another implant is inserted, some women rebound with extremely high estradiol levels. The estrogen spike, however, does not last long. Symptom-free intervals become shorter and shorter, and new implants become less and less effective. Another problem is that estradiol plasma levels can remain high for as long as three to four years after the implant has been removed. During that time, a woman would essentially be receiving unopposed estrogen (see p. XXX) unless she supplements progesterone.[16]

Developing a Spiritual Practice: Melding Inner and Outer Worlds

In the early part of this chapter, we explored hormones as messengers in the body. Miraculously this complex system of communication continues without any conscious attention on our part. Similarly communication passes to us, and sometimes through us, from the more subtle realms of spirit. Bringing our conscious attention to these whisperings from spirit can nurture our inner lives.

Earlier in this chapter, we discussed the most appropriate forms of hormones (if any) to support our physical bodies. Our inner, spiritual lives require the same careful consideration. At its best, spiritual practice deepens connection with God, Goddess, Creator, the Divine, All That Is, whatever you choose to name the core of your spirituality. Developing spiritual practice links us with the larger wheels, the circle of earth life as well and the circle of spirit, introduced in chapter 3. I think of this developing relationship as a "tending" process, like nurturing a garden or tending the hearth. If the seed of relationship is well tended, a plant may begin to grow that eventually vines into every aspect of your life. Instead of being an isolated time in your day, sitting on a cushion or a church pew, "spiritual practice" becomes a way of life that affects everything you do.

If you already have a spiritual practice, I would encourage you to ask the following questions as a way of deepening your practice. This "tending" is a lifelong process. As any gardener can attest, the "garden" is never complete.

Begin by asking the question, "What am I tending?" Keep in mind that the answer to that question may unfold slowly, like a tree gradually spreading its limbs at the edge of an open field.

Be patient. Allow your life to gestate a response to that query, "What am I tending?" With that answer firmly in your mind/heart, you can then ask, "How am I tending this relationship?"

The answers to these questions, if asked deeply and wholeheartedly, will vary for each of us. Reaching for handy responses from the catechism of your youth will not offer much sustenance now. Make space like an open field inside yourself to receive unexpected gifts. Plant those seeds, or allow the wind of spirit to navigate them into place. Tend these responses, for they are the seedbed of the next phase of your spiritual life.

Clarissa Pinkola Estes offers the hope, deeply rooted in her own tradition, of new life that comes from making the soil ready and patiently waiting for whatever will grow:

> *What is this faithful process of spirit and seed that touches empty ground and makes it rich again? Its greater workings I cannot claim to understand. But I know this: Whatever we set our days to might be the least of what we do, if we do not also understand that something is waiting for us to make ground for it, something that lingers near us, something that loves, something that waits for the right ground to be made so it can make its full presence known.*
>
> *I am certain that as we stand in the care of this faithful force, that what has seemed dead is dead no longer, what has seemed lost, is no longer lost, that which some have claimed impossible, is made clearly possible, and what ground is fallow is only resting— resting and waiting for the blessed seed to arrive on the wind with all Godspeed.[17]*

Fallow Fields

The "empty ground" Clarissa refers to seems to be a necessary prerequisite for profound transformation. A mentor once spoke of how any major life shift is preceded by a fallow period, when someone neither inhabits her previous life nor has navigated into the new. This "in-between" state could be likened to the caterpillar's transformation within the cocoon. As the cocoon hangs from a twig, nothing noteworthy is happening on the outside. Within those translucent walls, though, profound transformation is underway. The caterpillar cannot skip this stage and move immediately into life as a butterfly.

Similarly we cannot dramatically shift our inner orientation without a seemingly fallow outer period.

One participant at a meditation retreat shared his story of beginning a spiritual practice. He knew that he did not want to continue his life as it had been, but he had no idea how to change his life or what to change it into. For three months, he came home from work, ate dinner, sat on the sofa, and stared at the wall of his apartment.

"I literally stared at a blank wall," he recounted. "I didn't watch TV. I didn't call my friends. I didn't read books. I just sat there. And at the end of three months, I went to a meditation class. I really couldn't tell you why. I just knew I had to go. And I've never looked back. I still have the same job, but my friends, my activities, and my inner world are completely different."

The caterpillar probably could not explain why it has to spin a cocoon. It just *knows* it must. I offer you this story so you may recognize when you come to a similar crossroads in your life. Instead of chafing at these transitional periods, anxious to "get on with it," welcome these times of unknowing. Make space for the mystery to enter your life. Like the seed in winter ground, allow yourself to dream, to gestate new life within.

Gather Your Mentors

In chapter 3, I introduced the understanding of lineage and how direct contact with a teacher or mentor can usher us into a living tradition. I used to chafe at the suggestion that anyone seeking deep spiritual realization needed a teacher. Certainly many people reach profound realizations and live deeply spiritual lives without a human teacher or guide. Followers of all the great religions rely on the guidance of great teachers long after that savior or avatar has died. Having contact with a human teacher, however, allows the possibility of what might be best described as "transmission."

In many Asian traditions, teaching is passed experientially. As a qigong instructor, for example, I discovered that people who had learned qigong from a book or recording often missed important aspects of the practice. These students might still benefit from qigong practice, but their experience was incomplete. Imagine trying to drive a brand new truck that is missing one small component: the starter. Trying to engage a spiritual tradition without that primary "spark" of transmission is like trying to drive a truck that looks perfect on the outside but lacks vital inner components.

Mentors can help guide you in the "tending" process and offer valuable feedback. They can be especially helpful when you reach a dead end.

The Community of Spirit

Our hormones act as messengers that catalyze activity throughout the body. Hormones cannot act in isolation; they must literally attach to a cell wall and communicate with that structure to effect change. Hormones function within the larger cycles and systems of the body.

Cultivating a healthy spiritual practice also requires communication with outside sources. We need interaction with others to touch and be touched, to inspire and be inspired. Like a garden amended with com- posted manure and the previous season's fallen leaves, we need the nourish- ment of a larger circle to grow in healthy ways. A garden planted year after year without replenishing the soil eventually yields only weeds and stunted, bug-infested vegetables. Our individual soul, the smallest circle of life, needs the larger wheels of community and planetary life for healthy, sus- tainable growth.

Several years ago when I was living at the Findhorn Foundation in Scotland, I spent a week on the Isle of Iona. Traigh Bahn, the community's retreat house, was filled with summer guests, and I bunked with a dear friend who was the caretaker that summer. I was just beginning to consider leaving the community and moving on. . .to what? I had no idea where I was headed in my life.

One afternoon I entered the sanctuary with "The Game of Life," an orac- ular, transformational game developed at the Findhorn Foundation. I was hoping to receive guidance about next steps in my life. Playing alone, I even- tually moved into a place in the game known as "the dark night of the soul." I really *felt* the depths of that dark night. I sat in deep despair, wondering how I could move off this place on the board as well as within myself.

I sat in meditation for awhile, as I did not have any resources to con- tinue moving on the board. I gradually began to realize I did not have those resources within me either. As an individual, without the support of a com- munity or at least one other person, I could not move forward in my life. Late in the afternoon, my friend Jean came into the sanctuary, took a quick look at the pile of sodden tissues around me, and enveloped me in a hug.

"Judith, what are you doing?" she asked.

"I'm in the dark night of the soul." I broke into a fresh round of sobs.

"Oh, dearie, you can't be playing this by yourself. You're meant to play with other people. Here, let me join you."

With her patient support, I was able to move out of the dark night of the soul on the board. Eventually many friends and mentors, from both the seen and unseen realms, helped me literally move out of that dark night.

In retrospect, I realize my independent nature worked against me at that important juncture in my life. I had worked with the women who created "The Game of Transformation" and thought I had enough skill to navigate The Game on my own. That arrogant assumption haunted me as I realized the importance of the other "players" in my life.

If I was going to play The Game effectively, I couldn't be a lone cowgirl. Yes, I needed to tread my own path and listen to my own heart for guidance, but I needed community for reflection and sustenance on that journey.

Most spiritual traditions understand the importance of this larger sphere of support. In Buddhist traditions, practitioners "take refuge" in the sangha, the community of practice. That "community" includes the larger circle of all life as well as human society. In Christian traditions, we are reminded "God is first, my neighbor is second, and I am third." The gem in both of these traditions is the central importance of community to sustain our solitary practice. We are social animals, and mindful contact with others—especially at certain key points in our lives—can deepen our spiritual lives in ways that solitary practice alone cannot.

Tools for Tending the Garden

When asked what tools would best support women moving through menopause, Kathleen Luiten replies, "Meditate, meditate, meditate." Sharon Smith suggests, "Ritual, ritual, ritual." Both responses point toward powerful ways of developing, or deepening, our inner lives.

In chapter 12, we will look in depth at creating a celebration ritual to mark the menopausal passage. What Sharon refers to, though, is daily, ongoing communication with the Divine.

"Never go more than twelve hours without connecting with God, Goddess, Creator, whatever name you use," says Sharon. "That means having a morning and evening ritual, so that you are always close to spirit."

Rituals can take many forms. Much of our day is devoted to unconscious ritual, or habit: get up, use the toilet, put on shoes, scrub the sink, start breakfast, and so on. In this case, we are aiming at *consciously* creating ritual, applying keen observation to our daily tasks and inserting moments of deep connection into the rhythm of the day.

Washing dishes, for example, can be a profound ritual. Often I wash the dinner dishes after my boys have gone to sleep. "Om Tare, Tu Tare, Ture Swaha" runs through my mind as I fill the sink with water. "Om Tare, Tu Tare, Ture Swaha," I repeat silently as I squirt dishwashing liquid in the sink. "Om Tare, Tu Tare, Ture Swaha," I sing as I churn the dishes through the water. On evenings when I am frustrated or angry, I might invoke Quan Yin. If my frustration is beyond telling, I offer my troubles to Shiva's fire.

Many activities can become meaningful rituals. Below is a short list to spark your imagination. Allow yourself to be guided to the activities and rituals that most fully open you to spirit:

DANCING

Bernard Wosien, a twentieth-century ballet master, collected folk dances as he toured and performed in Europe. Over time, and through his own body experience, he discovered the Western mystery traditions embedded in these folk dances. Bernard's intuition told him that when the mystery traditions had to go underground, they were "hidden" in plain view, in the dances shared in the villages. He started a movement that is now known as "sacred dance." Bernard presented the folk dances as a way of experiencing the sacred mysteries directly through the body. The Dances of Universal Peace, from the Sufi tradition, reverently combine songs and movement. Gabrielle Roth pioneered spontaneous movements and dance as a profound path to healing and awakening. Move your body. Move your spirit. Both are intertwined.

SINGING

Every spiritual tradition incorporates sacred music. Singing and instrumental music literally change our vibratory rate. Sound, in the hands of an adept, can catalyze profound healing. The words of many sacred chants, especially from the Sanskrit and Latin, have the power to transform. Singing sacred songs can recalibrate us on all levels and deepen connection with the Divine.

Until the implementation of Vatican II, monks and nuns in Catholic monasteries sang "The Liturgy of the Hours." Monks and nuns gathered eight different times in a twenty-four-hour period to sing Gregorian chants, composed in special musical scales called "modes." These modal compositions can profoundly affect moods, thus opening one's ability to connect with the Divine. In the early 1960s, Vatican II instructed churches, nunneries, and monasteries to sing in the vernacular language. The Liturgy of the Hours was reduced from eight to seven services. Prayers replaced some of the singing. The modal Gregorian chants, developed over centuries, quickly began to disappear.

A priest I met years after this change described how the monks in his monastery had become very despondent at that time. The elders in the monastery brought in a consultant to help assess the change in the monks.

"What have you done differently in the last year?" the consultant asked. When he learned of the reduction in singing, the consultant wisely recommended they resume the former schedule of singing the Liturgy of the Hours in Latin. Within a month, the monks' depression had lifted.

MEDITATING

Meditation fine-tunes our ability to listen to body, mind, and spirit. During menopause, our bodies recalibrate on many levels. Part of the art of riding the rapids of menopause is learning to "gear up" or "gear down" our energy bodies. If we are stressed and the "heat rises" (often literally), we may need to gear up activity or mental focus. If we are lethargic and heavy, we may need to gear down, calm the mind and body, and slow our pace.

Meditation is the practice of being observant in the present moment. Notice—*be observant.*

"But my mind is so full of thoughts!" many people protest.

The point is not to be free of thoughts but rather to keep bringing the mind back to watchfulness. Our awareness "gains strength" by reining in our wandering thoughts.

Like wild horses, my mind tears off in many directions. "That fly reminds me of the Outback in Australia. I wonder what those two aboriginal girls are doing now, the ones with the wild hair, who took me out to show me lizard tracks among the rocks? The four-wheel drive Toyota truck we drove was just like my friend Sara's. Oh yeah, and I have to order the taillight for my car. Darn, I crunched the trunk on the corner of that truck in a parking lot last week. I hate those big, old, gas-guzzling trucks with titanium bumpers. What is that going to do to my insurance?

"Ah. Off track. Here. This moment. Breath moving in. Breath moving out. Breath moving in. Breath moving out. Gee, that clock is loud. I wonder what time it is? I wonder if the babysitter will be back by 4:15? Did I remember to leave dinner instructions? Oh, darn, I don't think I did. Will I have time to talk to her before dinner? I have to call. . .

"Ah. Breath. Here. Belly moving out. Belly moving in. Breath filling lungs. Breath moving out. Here. Silence."

The "strengthening" does not come from having a completely quiet mind, like a still pond on a moonlit night. The mental/spiritual muscle flexes and develops when I bring myself *back* to this moment. As those internal "muscles" strengthen over time, the periods of stillness become longer and more frequent. Those peaceful interludes, though, are not the goal of meditation but rather a side benefit.

Ramana Maharshi offers the following instructions for meditation:

> *You can use mantras, breath, or the quiet glow of a candle. Your technique is not important as long as you know this one simple thing: It is natural for thoughts to arise during meditation. You will say your mantra, then you will forget it as a wave of thoughts flow through. Then you say your mantra again. Simple as that. So, too, if you are meditating on your breath. You will feel your breathing, then you won't . . . because a herd of thoughts stampedes across your mind. This is perfectly natural. Perhaps that herd has been penned up for a long time. Thoughts long hidden within you arise when you meditate. Allow these thoughts to arise so they can dissolve in due time.*
>
> *Please ignore those well-meaning, earnest teachers—still trapped in the fascination and violence of their minds—who tell you to "stop" thought or "give up" attachments. They are merely trying to get you to do something they cannot do themselves. To try to stop your thoughts is like swatting at buffaloes. Amusing for the buffalo, a waste of effort for the swatter. Watch the buffalo stampede, then return to your mantra, return to your breath. No stampede lasts forever.[18]*

"But I don't have *time* to meditate!" I hear you say. Ironically, on the days when I meditate, I find my concentration and focus improve, allowing me to move more efficiently through the day. I more than make up the time I "wasted" in meditation.

You may ask in meditation to connect with the guide you met at the end of chapter 1. The more attention you pay to your guides and allies, the more support they can give you. This regular attention is similar to the process of "taking medicine" (albeit usually far more enjoyable)—most vitamins or drugs will help only if you remember to take them regularly!

I do not intend this chapter to be a primer on meditation. You can find many good books on the subject. Even better, find a teacher to mentor you in learning or deepening your meditation practice.

PRAYING

In meditation, I listen to spirit. In prayer, I speak to Creator. Gratitude is the foundation of prayer. Saints from many traditions have devoted themselves to prayerful appreciation of God's gifts. Many people also pray to request Creator's assistance.

My prayers have changed dramatically in the last decade. My sister's death just before her forty-first birthday uprooted my belief in a personal God. In retrospect, I'm not sure how this concept of a cozy fairy godmother/father developed. My sister's passing in combination with another tragedy later that year swept the remnants of a childhood God from my life. I suddenly understood that God does not stay up late at night worrying about the balance in my checking account. That is my job. Goddess is not plotting a career for me, repairing the roof, or inoculating my children against illness and tragedy. Creator had his/her own work and life to pursue: creating other worlds, playing golf, relaxing in a hot bath, whatever he/she wants to do.

When I recounted this realization to my Shawnee mentor, he nodded sagely. "Creator gave you life," he said, "and he, she, whatever you want to call it, gave you the ability to think and take care of yourself. That's your responsibility."

He paused for a moment, choosing his words carefully. "When I pray— and I do still pray—I ask for help in figuring something out. 'Creator, help me think through how to support my family. Help me figure out how to find a job.' You don't ask Creator to find the job for you or to give you the money. Life doesn't work that way. That would be insulting the intelligence Creator gifted you with. You pray as a capable person who needs help, not as a helpless human being."

The Shawnee medicine man's words still guide me in my prayers. I offer prayers of gratitude. I pray for loved ones' health and guidance. I also place healing requests into the Stream of Life, asking that each receives what he or she needs.

Search your own traditions for a deeper understanding of prayer. The path of prayer can open a profound connection with spirit.

WRITING IN A JOURNAL

Spending a few minutes in meditation and then writing in a journal can be deeply healing. *Writing as a Way of Healing* by Louise DeSalvo offers simple guidelines to evoke the deepest emotional healing from journal entries. The author suggests writing for twenty minutes a day, four days in a row. Make this commitment periodically so that you don't feel too overwhelmed at the prospect of having to write daily. The first chapter gives more specific dos and don'ts to gain the most benefit from your journal-writing practice.

Susan O'Toole, a gifted artist and qigong instructor in Ireland, found great support in journal writing during menopause:

What's my menopause all about?

Good question to begin with because it goes right to the heart of what it is, and what or who it's for. What purpose does it serve? Where does it begin and end? What's the relationship between it and you?

These are questions that kept coming back to me throughout the process, which did change and develop as we progressed together. It talks back to you as you go on. I realized that I could not push the process. I found it easier to cooperate. If ever I tried pushing the changes, to stop the resisting was uncomfortable, because it is bigger than us, and it's better not to get wrapped up too tightly about a natural occurrence.

I found as I went into the process, like going into the eye of a storm, I had an intimate, deep experience of being one with nature's cycles. I had a sense of reentering humanity in a new way, leaving the old behind and thus giving birth into the mystery of my own being.

I found it helpful to go and ask somebody if I was having night sweats or having sudden heat rushes. That somebody was a neighbor, friend, and strangers! I did keep a diary to talk through these changes. To me they became a series of transactions and interactions that were moving and alive, like life.

For those of you who are already in this extraordinary time of life

*or approaching the menopause, there isn't a right or wrong way of
what life should look like for you. Just be at home with yourself.
Enjoy exploring and journeying toward an understanding and discovering that the menopause is natural. It's an invitation to open to
the gift that we are.*

WALKING MEDITATION

This gentle, rhythmic movement can lead to deep, meditative states. For
some, sitting meditation is too constrained, dance too strenuous. For many,
walking is a comfortable middle way. Walking also offers the opportunity to
be outside, in connection with the earth. See Sylvia Boorstein's instructions
for classic walking meditation (p. XXX). If you find her instructions too
restrictive, simply walk with awareness and gratitude.

MAKING LOVE

Tantric sex is a pathway to the Divine. Truly making love, not just going
through the motions, can link us with the spark of the Divine within our
partner and ourselves. Mastering this physical expression of love can liberate
us to love all aspects of creation. See River Woman's comments about making love in chapter 7.

QIGONG

Most people begin to practice qigong to improve their health. Continued
practice benefits the spirit as well as the body. Learning to assimilate qi, or
vitality and life force, eventually links us to the Source of all life.

Embracing Formal Practices

For many, this life period is a time to learn or deepen a formal practice. You
may be drawn to learn sacred music or begin a chanting practice. The rosary
may call you to daily devotion. You may participate in silent retreats and
learn a specific meditation practice. You may feel called to serve a mission or
join a religious community.

In kabbalistic tradition, a man (or woman) does not study the kabbalah
until he is at least forty, married, with a family and a stable job. The Judaic
mystics understand that an earnest student needs to be skilled at living in
the physical world before pursuing the metaphysical realms. At this point in
your life, you likely have your feet firmly planted in the world. If you desire,

you are now ready to pursue more formal training, to send branches into other realms, and to become a channel between heaven and earth.

Allow your heart and soul to guide you to the practice(s) that deepen your relationship with spirit. Cultivating an attentive ear, discerning the whisperings of spirit, can ease the potential turmoil of this life transition. With practice, listening to the messages of spirit may become as effortless as the hormones' transmissions, catalyzing change on a soul, instead of a cellular, level.

Reflections by Sharon Jeanne Smith

Sharon Jeanne Smith lives as a lay Catholic monk in Santa Fe, New Mexico.

When perimenopause started for me in my early forties, I simply didn't know that was what was going on. I thought menopause was about periods ending and didn't know much at all about the perimenopause phase until after I lived through it and saw it written about later.

To give a little background about my own journey, I will just say that I was raised in a Protestant evangelical tradition that was devoid of all symbol and ritual—not a good match for me. The first time I ever walked into a Catholic church in 1960 when I was seventeen, I had an overwhelming mystical experience. It didn't have any perceptual content and what was going on at this pre–Vatican II service was not aesthetic in the least, but I was simply taken by love and never given back. I interpreted this as to become Catholic and that has served me well over the years. Needless to say, my family was rather dismayed at this decision, but I knew what my own truth was. In the ensuing years, I was in and out of the convent twice, knowing I wanted to give my life to God, but not finding convent living a good match for me. My alcoholic family background probably did not stand me in good stead for that communal life. I became a nurse and pursued graduate studies in nursing, theology, and philosophy. I had lots of energy, always did, and most of my learning was about how to focus and contain it. I was healthy and did not pay much attention to my body. In 1983, I completed my Ph.D. in philosophy and considered looking for work in academia.

I count my menopause journey as starting on December 8, 1983. On that day, I had an experience of watching my personal, social, and cultural constructions begin disintegrating before my very eyes. I had a Ph.D. in epistemology (the branch of philosophy that deals with what we can know and how we can know it) and knew that trying to build a new meaning system was futile since it would be a construction, just like the first one was, only I did not know it. I felt like life had lost all meaning, and I had been abandoned in a random universe—not a comfortable feeling! However, I intuitively knew that it was developmental, a stage in my development, and that I just had to let go into free fall and live in the moment and see what emerged. I decided not to make any changes in my life and continued to live and work where I was and just focus on living in the here and now.

In the spring, I started to pray what Catholics call the "office" again, officially called the Liturgy of the Hours. It is what monks and nuns have prayed for centuries, with or without chant, consisting mostly of psalms and scripture readings. The psalms convey just about every human emotion and predicament, and it was very helpful for me to pray them in the midst of my own darkness. The Catholic and Orthodox churches use all of the psalms in their liturgies, even the "smash 'em and bash 'em" ones that other churches leave out. It is useful to be able to connect with all aspects of our humanness during these kinds of times.

In the fall, I resumed going to church services. I had stopped five years previous to that because I could not tolerate the patriarchy in the Church. At about the age of thirty, I had finally figured out, with great relief and joy, that I was a lesbian and that did not help matters either. I returned knowing that I had to be true to myself in regard to my sexual preference, but also because I needed a container large enough to hold the process I was going through. And, while the Catholic Church is certainly patriarchal, it is also Mother Church and is a womb/caldron that holds all of the symbols and rituals that can aid me through transformation. I went to Mass three days in a row and the angst lifted. I was back in the place that could heal me.

About this time, I started to have psychic openings. I am not particularly psychic, although I am very intuitive about what I need and sometimes about what might be helpful to others. This opening came in the form of a tremendous empathic sensibility. If I went to a party—and I did love to go to parties and dance—I felt like everyone was a high-velocity fan blowing on me with their feelings. This was too much, and I significantly cut down on my social life. I was also easily irritated, which was hard on others, and they were happy for me to limit my social life. I had to become very conscious and choose carefully exactly what I would do, with whom, and how long. I think the greatest gift of menopause is the push to become conscious about and make choices about every minute of our time and every ounce of our energy.

A year or two later, I decided to leave my job and move to Santa Fe. The first year was difficult since I did not really know how I was to proceed. An attempt to continue in the same vein professionally met with a stone wall, and I needed to find simple work, first in nursing. About a year later, I left nursing completely and started to work part-time doing secretarial tasks and cleaning. I am particularly good at putting and keeping things in order and have supported myself that way ever since.

I call this period of my life a time of "being undone." It was a break from my previous life and the start of becoming who I am now. Not long after I moved to Santa Fe, I had an eruption of kundalini energy, with lots of body energetics happening. Needless to say my Catholic background didn't give me much information on these goings on. I found books that were helpful, mostly in the Hindu tradition, and a woman healer who could help manage the energetics, but who could not teach me how to do it myself. It took a couple of years for all of this to calm down. If I got the least bit off center, then my energy would erupt. I was on a short leash and soon learned to hold my center—or else. I was in half a meditative state half the time for about two years and this kept me in silence and solitude a lot.

I also could not do much in the way of heavy intellectual reading or thinking. I started to read lives of the saints, of all kinds and traditions— saints are saints. I sought for commonalties that crossed traditions, cultures, and historical periods. I found this very helpful. When the cults of the saints began to arise in Christianity during the sixth century, they were called "invisible friends," and they were indeed that for me, true fellow travelers on this rather bumpy journey.

I also used my Catholic practices to good advantage. I found a priest who really knows how the Sacrament of Reconciliation (confession) is truly a healing sacrament. When I became aware of a psychological pattern that needed to be let go, I went to confession to him and that pattern would indeed dissipate. I love the sacraments, they're free and they work! I also used the Sacrament of the Sick if some pattern was hardwired into my nervous system. If I was working on a particular pattern, I would remember it at the beginning part of the Mass during what is called the penitential rite and then when I received communion later would see it as true medicine to heal that pattern.

I began to really work consciously with each decision during my day, honing my intuition to know what I was "supposed" to do. In the beginning of this, I would literally ask myself about everything—should I get up, should I go to the bathroom, should I go to work, and so on. This helped me to get adept at making conscious choices and staying open to however my life was to develop. I was financially quite poor during this time, but I did get everything I needed, although it was not always easy.

At this time, I looked seriously at who I really was. I realized that I am really a monk, and I am not supposed to live in a monastery. I had never formed a partner relationship that I wanted to be permanent. God had become my primary partner during that experience when I was seventeen, and I found that nothing and no one had ever been able to match it. I made private vows and began to live a lay monastic life very seriously.

I finally looked closely at my alcoholic family background and began to go to Adult Children of Alcoholics (ACA) meetings. I found this very helpful and was able to identify the patterns that continued to run my life unconsciously and to work with them with the Catholic sacraments as I described above. Physically I had a number of perimenopausal symptoms during this time. I was tired a lot, had ferocious headaches that were not migraines but seemed to be tied to approaching storms, which we have every afternoon during the summer monsoon season here in New Mexico, and I had terrible insomnia. Someone suggested that I just forget about ever sleeping again, and that was actually helpful. I was working part-time and did have time to rest during the day if I needed to.

I also started to cry easily. It didn't have anything to do with being sad or angry, but anytime something touched me, I cried. I stopped watching the news; the images were simply too overwhelming. I still do not watch the news and still cry easily when touched, but it has improved over the years.

A couple of years after I moved to Santa Fe, I got the intuition to sell everything and go to Europe. I did this and set out with $600 in my pocket. I landed penniless in Rome ten days later. A circumstance took me to Assisi where I lived for a few months with Tenzin Palmo, an English Tibetan Buddhist nun. I then lived with other American and English families for five months. I was up against all my security fears during this time and learned experientially that I always had what I needed. Again, this was not easy, but it taught me that I am "always held," and I no longer have fears about my security.

I returned to the United States and went to Denver for six months of more living on the financial edge and then knew that I could move on from there. A friend who had just retired invited me to come to California and stay with her for a while and help her put all of her files, closets, and so on in order. I did this and began my "maid monk" career for the next six years, staying with friends and being their maid half the time and a monk the rest of the time. I had no income nor personal space and learned to let go of a number of needs to be in control. It was during this time that my period stopped as I turned fifty. Then I began to have hot flashes, though mild. I learned to be careful of caffeine, alcohol, and garlic if I did not want to trigger them. My headaches continued, and I developed psoriasis of the hands.

In 1995, I decided it was time to settle down again, to live alone, and to foster my spiritual journey with more silence and solitude. I moved back to Santa Fe and now support myself doing personal assistant work. I live simply in one room with a limited wardrobe and no car. I have five-day weekends and take at least four weeks off a year for retreats, both at a woman's Benedictine monastery where I am affiliated as an Oblate and here in my tiny, baby monk cell with its eighteen-inch-thick adobe walls. As a gregarious extrovert, this semi-hermit lifestyle was somewhat of a surprise, but I find I am very happy in it. I entered this journey a very busy professional and came out the other end a lay monk living a very contemplative life.

My own Roman Catholic tradition was most helpful during the menopausal period of my life. The crucifixion-resurrection is all about the possibility of transformation at any moment under any circumstance for everyone if they will open up to it. The sacramental system, symbols, and rituals are a real help to me, I resonate with them immediately and they guide me deeper and deeper. I was not raised Catholic and was not taught some very poor theology as a child, which unfortunately happened to many who were raised Catholic. I have a fine graduate theological education and have read extensively in the very broad Catholic tradition giving me access to much that is beyond what one might find in a typical parish. The doctrine of the Trinity, which seems like so much confusion to many, is really about the Divine being by nature relatedness, and that reality itself is relatedness and nonseparation. Knowing this at a deep level leads to more and more compassion for myself and others.

You may contact Sharon Jeanne Smith at: 1202 Cerro Gordo Road, Santa Fe, New Mexico 87501   Can 1 line be cut from this page?

CHAPTER FIVE

PHYTOESTROGENS: HERBAL KNOWLEDGE and HEALING WISDOM

PHYTO MEANS "PLANT," SO *PHYTOESTROGENS* ARE PLANT MOLECULES THAT mimic estrogen's activity in the body. They can bind at estrogen receptor sites, but their effect is much weaker than the estrogens we make. Most phytoestrogens, for example, are one hundred to one thousand times weaker than estradiol, the strongest-acting endogenous estrogen.[1]

PLANT-BASED ESTROGENS AND HOW THEY WORK

Phytoestrogens can either increase or decrease overall estrogen activity. How could one substance have two seemingly opposite functions? A phytoestrogen's "strength" or effect depends on its affinity for certain tissue receptors (for example, breast vs. endometrium), the amount, the type of phytoestrogen, and overall estrogen levels in the body. To explain the last factor, I use the analogy of a movie theater.

Phytoestrogens Go to Hollywood

Imagine that every seat in a movie theater is an estrogen-receptor site. Let's say that 100 percent–filled seats would represent normal reproductive-age estrogen levels. During menopause, how many of the seats would be filled? (If you need to review, see chapter 3.) Estrogen drops 40 to 60 percent by the beginning of menopause (one year with no menstrual bleeding), so the theater seats would be about half filled.

In this case, if a perimenopausal or menopausal woman was experiencing minor estrogen deficiency symptoms such as mild hot flashes, night sweats and/or vaginal dryness, she might consider supplementing phytoestrogens. The weaker phytoestrogens would not try to muscle the body's stronger estrogens out of their seats. Instead, the phytoestrogens would "sit" in the empty seats, filling the empty receptor sites and thereby increasing overall estrogen activity.

Consider another scenario: a forty-four-year-old woman suffering with fibrocystic breasts, mood swings, bloating, irritability, and heavy menstrual bleeding. She has a host of estrogen dominance symptoms. If 100 percent–filled seats was normal, in her situation the theater would probably be packed to capacity—standing room only with estrogens spilling into the aisles, lobby, and out the front door.

In this case, you may think to yourself, "This woman already has far too much estrogen. Why would she want to add phytoestrogens?" Remember that phytoestrogens are much weaker than the estrogens our bodies produce. Phytoestrogens can join the crowd of estrogens (and possibly xenoestrogens) in the aisles, waiting for a seat to open. Usually an estrogen molecule "sits" in a receptor site for three to six hours (about long enough for a double feature!) before unbinding and reentering the bloodstream.

When a seat opens, the phytoestrogens, endogenous estrogens, and xenoestrogens compete to fill the empty seat. Of course the phytoestrogens will not win a seat every time. Eventually, though, if we maintain a steady supply of phytoestrogens, perhaps 5 or 10 percent of the seats will fill with phytoestrogens. With some seats occupied by phytoestrogens, do you think overall estrogen activity would go up or down? Remember that the phytoestrogens are much weaker, so overall estrogen activity decreases.

Consider Japanese women who eat a significant amount of soy, a major food source of phytoestrogens. These women have phytoestrogens in the "aisles" all the time. Although Japanese women probably produce as much endogenous estrogen, their overall estrogen activity tends to be lower than Western women who do not consume the same volume of phytoestrogens. Lowered estrogen activity could at least in part explain why Japanese women tend to be at lower risk for breast and other reproductive cancers. Unfortunately when Japanese women abandon their traditional diet and adopt Western eating habits, their risk for developing breast cancer quickly rises to match Western women's.

Because a woman eating a traditional Japanese diet is accustomed to lower overall estrogen activity, the shift into menopause probably will not be as dramatic for her. In addition, she continues to have phytoestrogens in the "aisles" to fill the emptied seats/receptor sites. Her estrogen activity remains much more constant during this menopausal transition than her Western counterparts.

Can I Replace My Prescription Estrogen with Phytoestrogens?

After learning about phytoestrogens, many women ask if they can eat phytoestrogen-rich foods and herbs instead of taking prescription estrogen. The simple answer is "No," because the phytoestrogens are so much weaker. Even eating huge platefuls of tofu several times a day could not replace the estrogen activity of prescribed bio-identical or "conjugated" (horse) estrogens. Women who require estrogen—for example, to treat severe osteoporosis and/or severe menopausal symptoms—need to continue taking their estrogen prescription.

Phytoestrogen Foods

For women with mild bone loss and/or mild to moderate menopausal symptoms, phytoestrogens offer a terrific treatment option. Because of their weaker hormonal signal, phytoestrogens can help reduce estrogen-dominance symptoms in perimenopausal women. As you learned in the analogy above, they bind to receptor sites so that the stronger estrogens have fewer places to "sit." Phytoestrogens may also have a protective effect on breast tissue because they block stronger estrogens from binding and "whisper" instead of shout their hormonal messages.

THE JOY OF SOY

Soy foods such as tofu, tempeh, soy milk, and cooked soybeans contain isoflavones that have phytoestrogenic activity. Whole soybeans have the highest isoflavone content, 1 to 2 mg per gram of soy protein. If you are using a soy powder or capsule, check the isoflavone content on the label.

Nutritional researchers suggest that Japanese women's low breast- and colon-cancer rates and rare incidence of hot flashes and other menopausal symptoms are related to their high soy protein intake.[2, 3] Western women consuming 160 mg of soy isoflavones daily for three months had significant reduction in hot flashes and vaginal dryness.[4] Women supplementing only 40 mg of soy isoflavones per day for twelve weeks had less dramatic results, with only minor reduction in hot flash symptoms.[5]

In addition to reducing menopausal symptoms, soy protects against cardiovascular disease by lowering total cholesterol, LDL cholesterol, and triglycerides.[6] Animal studies suggest soy may inhibit bone loss[7], but we have no long-term human studies to verify this effect in humans. Soy reduces the risk of developing breast[8, 9, 10] as well as endometrial cancer.[11] Eating other foods containing phytoestrogens—for example, whole grains, vegetables, seaweeds, fruits, and fiber—also lowers risk of endometrial cancer.[12]

Optimal Amounts of Soy Isoflavones for Menopausal Women

We have no definitive answer about how much soy to include in your diet to optimize health. I would suggest approximating the amount of soy products and soy isoflavones in a traditional Japanese diet, that is, 50 to 150 mg of soy isoflavones per day.

Keep in mind that more is not necessarily better. Eating too much tofu, from Chinese perspective, "cools" the digestive tract, giving rise to more gas and bloating. Many people are sensitive or outright allergic to soy. In fact, soy is one of the top ten food allergens in the United States. For women who are sensitive or allergic to soy, choose other phytoestrogens for support.

FLAXSEEDS AND LIGNANS

Flaxseeds contain more lignans, another class of phytoestrogens, than any other food. In addition to phytoestrogen activity, lignans have antitumor and antioxidant effects.[13, 14, 15, 16] Flaxseeds are also one of the only food sources of linolenic acid, an essential fatty acid.

Whole flaxseeds, flaxseed flour, and defatted flax meal are your best sources of lignans. Flax oil contains very little of the lignans. You can add whole flaxseeds to cooked breakfast cereal or blend them with "smoothies." Sprinkle flax meal on salads or over steamed vegetables.

Recommended Use: Aim for 1 to 2 tablespoons of whole flaxseeds or flax meal per day.

PHYTOESTROGEN HERBS FOR MENOPAUSAL WOMEN

Some women cannot eat soy products, either because of digestive problems or a soy allergy. Fortunately we have other options for supplementing phytoestrogens.

Black Cohosh (*Cimicifuga racemosa*)

Probably one of the most studied phytoestrogen herbs, black cohosh has a long history of use for menopausal symptoms. Like soy products, black cohosh reduces hot flashes in many menopausal women. Black cohosh probably reduces hot flashes by binding at estrogen receptor sites and lowering pituitary leutenizing hormone (LH) secretion.[17]

Animal studies suggest that black cohosh inhibits the breakdown of bone. As with soy, we have no human studies to confirm this information.[18] Black cohosh can help alleviate depression and increase vaginal wall thickness and lubrication.[19]

Recommended Use: 1 to 2 capsules or tablets twice a day (40 mg standardized extract) or $1/2$ to 1 teaspoon of standardized liquid extract. At this dose level, most women can take black cohosh long term without any problems.

Chaste tree berry (*Vitex agnus castus*)

Although this herb has often been recommended for menopausal symptoms, chaste tree berry affects progesterone more than estrogen levels. Chaste tree berry increases LH secretion, which in turn favors progesterone production. Remember LH can only promote progesterone production in the ovary if a woman is still ovulating.

Dong Quai (*Angelica sinensis*)

In Chinese medicine, dong quai is classified as a yin and blood builder. The Chinese view many menopausal symptoms as the result of diminished "yin" in the body. In their more poetic description of the body, the Chinese define yin as the moisturizing, nourishing, cooling properties in the body. By the time of menopause, most of us have severely depleted yin stores as a result of diet, stress, excessive thinking, too much activity, and too little rest. Think of yin as the cooling fluid in a car radiator. Without enough coolant, the radiator overheats. Extending the analogy to the human body, too little yin leads to a host of heat-related symptoms, for example, hot flashes, night sweats, headaches, dry skin, and dry hair.

Dong quai helps restore yin and blood, thereby reducing many heat-related symptoms. In Chinese medicine, dong quai would not be prescribed alone. A practitioner trained in Chinese herbs almost always prescribes herbs in combination, not as single agents. During a twelve-week study in the United States, women who supplemented dong quai alone did not have significant reduction in hot flashes, measurable changes in vaginal cells, or increased uterine lining thickness. Researchers concluded that dong quai had no estrogen-like activity in the body.[20] In this case, scientists incorrectly assumed that dong quai's effects were related to hormone-like activity and tested that hypothesis using Western pharmacological methods.

The Chinese prescribe herbs with a different understanding of herb functions and actions. If you want maximum benefit from dong quai and other Chinese herbs, I would recommend working with someone trained in prescribing Chinese herbal formulas rather than self-medicating.

CAUTION: Dong quai increases menstrual flow and can bring on menses. If you are perimenopausal and already suffer from heavy menstrual bleeding, dong quai probably is not the herb of choice for you.

Ginseng (*Panax ginseng*)

Korean and Chinese ginseng contain ginsenosides, compounds that have a variety of actions in the body. Ginseng can reduce mental or physical fatigue,[21] support the adrenal glands,[22] and increase vaginal wall thickness and lubrication.[23]

The Chinese classify Korean and Chinese ginsengs as warming herbs that build "qi" (or "chi") increasing overall energy and well-being. American ginseng (Panax quinquifolium) is both a qi and yin tonic, that is, it builds the nourishing, cooling properties and boosts vital energy. If you supplement Korean (the "hottest") or Chinese ginseng and notice an increase in heat-related symptoms, you may want to switch to American ginseng.

Recommended Use: 4 to 6 grams per day of powdered ginseng root. If you are using standardized extract capsules, supplement 200 mg per day of 5 percent ginsenoside or 100 mg per day of 10 percent ginsenoside.

PHYTOESTROGENS FOR MENOPAUSAL WOMEN

Just as with the prescription hormones, use phytoestrogen herbs only if you have a specific need such as hot flashes or vaginal dryness. Soy and flaxseeds, however, have health-promoting benefits in addition to their phytoestrogen effects that can support your overall health during this menopausal transition.

HEALING WISDOM: DEEPENING YOUR KNOWLEDGE OF HERBS

As recently as a century ago, many people had the good fortune of living in communities where grandmothers, uncles, medicine people, and healers worked with the ancient wisdom of plants. Today many interested in "natural" or "alternative" medicine are in the process of rediscovering this deeply rooted knowledge. I offer you the following insights to encourage you in that process of discovery. You are embarking on a journey that could last a lifetime. These four steps are common guideposts I have witnessed in my own and others' learning process.

1. "Use This for That."
   Many people accustomed to seeking conventional medical help are trained to think in terms of one medicine to treat one ailment. Prilosec treats stomach acid, for example, and Prozac treats depression. Take this to treat that. Those beginning to experiment with herbs, homeopathics, and nutritional supplements usually bring this same mentality to using natural medicines, for example, take comfrey to heal bones; use St. John's Wort for depression.

   Few beginners understand that effectively choosing a homeopathic or a botanical medicine requires a completely different paradigm. "Natural," or what I prefer to call "classical," medicine views the *person* who is suffering with a particular condition, rather than a *disease* affecting a particular body. Conventional medicine simply looks at the disease and prescribes this drug to treat that disease. Classical medicine treats the person who is suffering with a disease. Ten different people with the same medical diagnosis, for example, might take ten different homeopathic remedies or ten different combinations of herbs to address their particular set of symptoms.

   A common misunderstanding in this first stage of exploration is that only pharmaceutical drugs qualify as "medicine." One day while waiting in line at the post office, I happened to meet a patient who had come to me for help with menopausal symptoms several months before. "Oh, that's all taken care of," she explained to me. "I went to my medical doctor for some medicine." As I left the post office, I wondered to myself what she thought the hormones and herbs I had prescribed were. If they were not "medicine," were they "candy" or "placebos"? Perhaps I had failed in explaining to her that these substances were indeed potent medicines, albeit ones that might take some time to address the hormonal changes she was experiencing. Many people are accustomed to the lightening-quick action of pharmaceutical drugs. The primary aim of these drugs, however, is to override, not support, the body's innate healing processes. Patients may not understand that some natural substances require time to rebalance the body. Of course some natural medicines can act very quickly, as anyone who has used homeopathic arnica for a badly bruised knee or twisted ankle can verify.

Many natural health-care practitioners also rely on the "this for that" model when prescribing natural medicines. One of my former office partners worked for several years as a pharmaceutical company representative before entering chiropractic school. In her practice, she prescribed many supplements using the same pharmaceutical paradigm. She simply substituted supplements for drugs. "Here, take this for sleep. Take that for sore muscles. Take this for indigestion." She did not understand the importance of balancing nutrients (for example, always combining calcium with magnesium, or prescribing all of the B-vitamins together rather than in isolation) or tailoring prescriptions for individual patients. Why, for example, was the patient having trouble sleeping? Was depression an underlying issue? Did the patient eat well, including plenty of B-vitamin-rich whole grains? Did she exercise? Did muscle spasms keep her awake? These concerns were never considered. Most of her patients improved some with her prescriptions, but they did not experience the full potential benefit of the herbs or supplements.

2. Functions and Actions of Herbs.
In this second stage, a student of natural medicine begins to delve into the way a particular herb or nutrient works in the body. Comfrey promotes tissue healing, for example, because it contains a substance called "allantoin" that stimulates cell division. Plants are conglomerates of many elements with numerous different actions.

"Standardized" preparations of herbs focus on one specific substance in a plant, assuming that one particular element governs the effect of that plant. In truth, though, this is another shading of the "this for that" mentality. No one substance "rules" the action of a plant. Many elements contribute to the way a plant influences our bodies. This complexity explains why a single plant might be prescribed for many different reasons. Today St. John's Wort is most commonly prescribed for depression. Twenty years ago, though, St. John's Wort was mainly used for nerve damage and nervelike pain. As a topical oil (applied to the skin), St. John's Wort treats burns, sciatic pain, and crush injuries (again related to its effect on the nervous system).

The functions and actions of an herb are discovered through scientific research. Most cutting-edge herbal research is conducted in Germany, where they still have a centuries-old unbroken tradition of using plants as medicine.

3. Energetics of Herbs.

Discovering the energetic properties of herbs requires stepping outside the Western scientific paradigm and relying on ways of knowing not easily recorded by machines. Chinese herbalists in particular have pioneered this branch of botanical medicine over nearly six thousand years of continuous practice. The energetic attributes of herbs include such properties as heating, drying, cooling, tonifying, and moistening. In Chinese herbalism, plants are classified according to actions, for example, herbs that "dry dampness" or "clear toxic heat" or "nourish the blood." Herbs are also grouped according to the internal organs they affect. Rather than relying on guesswork, this information was gleaned by people who had the ability to "see" subtle energetic changes in the body. When someone ingested a particular herb, the sensitive person would "see" a particular organ or acupuncture channel associated with that organ "light up." We do not have scientific instruments in the West that can duplicate these ways of knowing. From my perspective, lacking such machines does not invalidate the information, but rather highlights the limitations of our current Western technology.

Western herbalism also has a historical tradition of identifying energetic properties of herbs. In the Middle Ages, herbalists commonly discussed these energetic actions. Some of that information has passed by word of mouth and written documents into modern times.

Prescribing herbs according to energetic principles requires evaluating the whole person, not just the disease. In Chinese medicine, a practitioner gathers information by asking questions, checking tongue and pulses, and then developing a "syndrome picture" that describes the patient's condition from an energetic perspective that is rooted in a deep understanding of organ functions. The Chinese herbalist does not prescribe herbs for a particular "disease;" instead she chooses herbs to treat the syndrome picture, which is gleaned from examining the whole person.

4. Essence or Spiritual Properties of Herbs.

One of my beloved teachers was a Chippewa (Anishnabe) man named Sun Bear. His people recognize three major healing traditions within their nation: those who heal by sharing wisdom, those who heal with their hands, and those who heal with herbs. He considered himself mainly a wisdom-healer, but Sun Bear also had a formidable knowledge of herbs and other healing techniques. During a break in one of his teachings, a woman approached Sun Bear to ask him about the healing properties of a particular herb. Sun Bear paused for a moment and looked quizzically at the woman. "You're a two-legged, just like me," he said finally. "Why don't you go ask the plant?"

Sun Bear was describing an ability that I believe most, if not all, humans possess: the ability to quiet our minds and listen deeply to other elements of creation. Plants, animals, rocks, and water are continuously communicating with each other and with us humans. Most of us, though, are too distracted with the busyness of our lives to quiet our minds enough to truly listen. I offer you these simple exercises to initiate the process of deep listening.

DEEP LISTENING EXPERIENCE

Choose a plant that draws you, catches your eye, or interests you because of its healing attributes. Seat yourself in front of the plant and allow your eyes to focus softly on the plant. Take a few deep breaths and visualize your thoughts drifting away like clouds blown on a breezy spring day. As you relax, imagine you are breathing the very essence of that plant into your heart. Allow your heart to expand and soften until you sense the essence of that plant rooting right in the center of your being. Sit quietly, allowing the plant to share any of its wisdom with you. This "knowledge" may come in the form of words, images, or a quiet knowing that stretches beyond words. Gradually draw your focus back to yourself and the place where you are sitting. Write or draw any impressions you receive from the plant.

If you enjoy drawing and artwork, you can experiment with a variation of the exercise above. Place paper, pencils, pens, and any other art supplies you may need in front of you. Sit quietly with a plant or flower, gazing with "soft focus" (slightly blurry vision). Breathe the essence of the plant into your heart. With your eyes still softly focused on the plant or flower, pick up a pencil or paintbrush, and begin to move your hand over the paper. Allow the plant's essence to guide your hand. You are aiming to portray the "soul" of the plant, its divine essence, not a literal interpretation of the plant's outer form. Continue relaxing, breathing in the plant's essence, as your hand moves over the paper.

You may choose to repeat these exercises over time. Each experience will draw you deeper and deeper into the spiritual essence of plants. The information you receive may surprise you. One friend who tried the first exercise with dandelion later researched the plant's healing properties in several herbal books. "I was shocked," she reported. "The books only scratched the surface. The plant had so much more to say!"

Reflections by Dr. Janet Scavarda

Dr. Scavarda grew up in rural Illinois growing almost everything she ate. Her relationship with plants goes back as far as she can remember. During her twenties, while working in commercial greenhouses, she began studying plants, particularly medicinal herbs. After graduating from chiropractic college and establishing her own practice, Dr. Scavarda began to incorporate plant medicines, emotional-release techniques, and aromatherapy into her practice. After moving to Grand Junction, Colorado, Dr. Scavarda reduced her practice to part-time, became a registered aromatherapist, and began teaching aromatherapy classes. She currently lives in Montrose, Colorado.

My journey into menopause began before any physical manifestations were noted, before I even remotely suspected it was happening. It began with a desire to put my life in order, to make changes that I had needed to make but had long delayed in order to raise my child, produce income, and keep my relationship intact.

As women, we often make a lot of trade-offs in life, put up with many things in our relationships, careers, and lives to keep things running smoothly. We put our lives on hold, put our aspirations aside, and try to keep all of the balls in the air for everyone else through the "raising the family" years. Often we lose ourselves for a time. Menopause is often when we begin to find ourselves again.

For me, menopause brought about the most profound and disconcerting changes of my life. The first thing I noticed was the inability, or flat-out refusal, to tolerate any aspect of my life that made me unhappy or diminished who I felt I was. My husband had cause to use the time-honored refrain, "It never bothered you before!" The often-used retort, "Well, it bothers me now!" was not truly accurate. It (whatever it was) had always bothered me; I had just let it slide for a myriad of peacekeeping, choose-your-battles reasons. My son was out of the house, I was wiser, and in every situation I sought happiness rather than strife. During this second half of my life, I was less willing to compromise my happiness; I knew it colored my future and determined the success of my relationships.

My brain chemistry, my hormones, my body, my spirit, and my emotions were all pushing me to stop being who was accepted by the external world and start being the person that I knew I was born to be. I spent the first part of my life nurturing and observing—my child as he grew, my marriage as it progressed, evolving family relationships, and my beloved patients. I say "beloved" patients because, over the years, I have learned the most from them. In their quest for health, they opened their lives to me, and I am forever in their debt.

In chiropractic college, I was taught, among other things, how to treat neck pain and headaches. But what I wasn't taught, and learned very quickly, was that finding and acknowledging the underlying emotional component was often as important as the treatment. For instance, knowing that the patient was going through a divorce and was financially or emotionally stressed allowed other avenues for treating the pain that brought them to me. We could discuss this kind of life change, how it was affecting them physically: jaw clenching, shoulders up to their ears, fear that was causing digestive problems. And we could address the most important fact for their well-being: that their current pain and dysfunction were temporary, that it was mirroring their current life situation, and that I was their resource for physical support through this time. You cannot change what you do not acknowledge. They were now able to supplement my care with other forms of support like massage, stress reduction, counseling, use of essential oils, hot baths, yoga, weight lifting, breathing techniques, whatever eased or balanced the current multilevel situation. This held true for everyone: mom with a migraine headache and heartburn, attorney with neck pain and hypertension, construction worker with low-back pain. Physical treatment in combination with life management was the winning combination. Sometimes physical resolution of a health problem cannot occur without resolving a contributing emotional or stress-related issue.

Fortunately for me, I entered menopause armed with this information. The "symptoms," at least in my case, were emotional and spiritual before they became physical. When the symptoms did become physical, I wasn't searching for the panacea herb or hormone. I knew that it didn't exist. I would need to address this new stage of my life in a multitude of ways from diet and exercise

to personal fulfillment and addressing the issues that my emotions were asking me to resolve. I utilized many tools on a physical level to assist the menopausal transition, but in the end, nothing helped more than happiness, than reaching the end of the day with a sense of fulfillment.

Menopause has been a slow awakening into this new stage of my life. Adjustments had to be made, and I learned that it was better to embrace them rather than fight them. Alchemical happenings—something in our brains, our bodies, and our consciousness, moves us forward. I believe it is the natural order of things to evolve and move forward. As is true in any area of life, resistance to forward movement always brings pain and discomfort. Complacency breeds stagnation and discomfort prods change. Menopause is not some terrible, hormonal mistake that curses women. I believe it is by the design of the Creator that at this time in our lives we are provided an opportunity to transform ourselves. Contrary to popular belief and all outward appearances, I did not go crazy during menopause; I became sane.

Before I entered menopause, I wish I had known that it was a continuing, incredibly individual process. No one thing works for everyone physically, mentally, spiritually, or emotionally. And what works for an individual initially may not work three, six, or nine months down the road. As I transitioned through the process, a number of different things worked for a period of time, but as I changed, the things that balanced me had to change as well.

My first physical manifestations of menopause were night sweats and insomnia. I found a combination of soy foods and essential oil of clary sage minimized and eventually eliminated this problem. I would either drink a cup or two of soymilk during the day, or I would start out the day with a smoothie made of tofu and fruit. At night, I would put a drop or two of medicinal-grade essential oil of clary sage on a tissue and place it on my pillow and breath the relaxing, hormone-balancing aroma as I went to sleep.

At about the same time, I had moved to a new city and was starting a new practice. I was arranging my practice so that I had more time to spend with patients (what I loved about my work) and less frustrating paperwork (what I disliked about my work). I was also making wonderful new friends with similar interests a shared perspective on life. We were great personal support for each other, and I felt like I was blossoming. The winning combination: addressing physical needs while making life changes that brought me happiness. For several months, menopausal symptoms abated and peace ensued.

Several months later, however, I began to have long, nearly hemorrhaging menstrual periods. I had never experienced anything like this in my life. They were leaving me weak and depleted, and sometimes it would only be a week or ten days before the next one started. At the same time, I was also developing vaginal dryness in between periods that was making intercourse less than enjoyable. I had just become a registered aromatherapist, and I was starting to teach aromatherapy classes. I had been hearing about research that was being done on an essential oil called *Vitex agnus castus* and its usefulness in mitigating menopausal symptoms. Chaste tree berry, its common name, had been used for centuries for reproductive maladies. Unlike the herbal form, which was made from the berries, this was an essential oil distilled from the leaves of the plant.

I obtained some *Vitex* essential oil from a friend of mine who had a small essential oil business. I began using it right after one of those horrible menstrual periods. I applied it topically to my abdomen every one or two days and was quite pleased to notice a change in my vaginal tissue within about two weeks, no more dryness. I also went the usual full month before my next period began, which was bad by my usual standards, but not quite as long and miserable as before using the *Vitex.* I had one more period after that, and I haven't had one since. That was about two and a half years ago. I continued using the *Vitex* for a few months after my last period and then gradually discontinued its use.

By this time, I had begun teaching aromatherapy classes, something I loved to do. I also started a monthly women's group with new friends and other health-care professionals. We would get together monthly, discuss fascinating topics, encourage and support each other, and eat delectable good-ies. I was also attending to a healthy diet and regular exercise routine.

My next adventure through menopause came as the much discussed hot flashes. As I read more literature, I began to pay more attention to my diet. I came to see a direct correlation between my sugar consumption and the onset and frequency of my hot flashes. I didn't quite eliminate sugar from my diet altogether, but I made a substantial reduction. As I expected, there was a correlating reduction in the number of hot flashes that I was experi-encing. And, of course, there remains the one constant that I have experi-enced throughout menopause: constant change, new stirrings, evolution.

It has been eight years since my first menopausal experiences, and the journey continues. What I can tell you about this time in my life is that I am healthier and happier than I was when it all began. I also think I am living more of my potential than ever before. I know more about who I am and what I want, and I have made some of the closest friendships of my life. I will not deny that I have had to move though much discomfort; certainly physically and most definitely emotionally and spiritually, but I like where I am. If it took menopause to get me here, that is fine; I am all the better for it.

Janet Scavarda, DC, 9017 Harvard Court, Montrose, CO 81401; (970) 323-5971

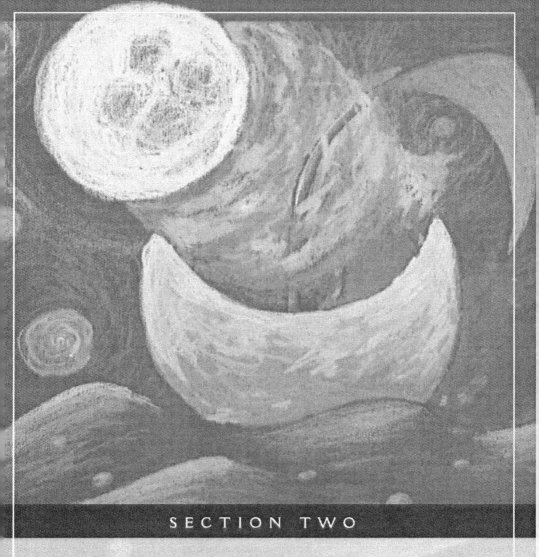

ENTERING the RAPIDS

Prelude to Section 2

The canoe gains speed in the current. The water is beginning to swirl, and River Woman digs her paddle into the water. I grip my paddle tighter. The river suddenly gives way beneath us, and we drop into whitewater and foam—nothing solid, just movement.

The river runs smoothly for a few yards and then drops again. We fly with the spray down a short waterfall. When we land, the canoe transforms into a kayak.

"The vehicle must be appropriate to the terrain," shouts the woman, her brown tunic drenched with water. Something more modern, I think to myself. Something sleek and hard and fast.

"You have to go with the flow when the water becomes this wild," she advises.

I sense myself drifting upward, moving away from the turbulent rapids and watching our progression from above.

"No. You have to be here," she explains quickly, digging a paddle into a rapid to avoid a boulder. "Focus on what is right in front of you. Work. The kids. Practice. You have to be right in the moment to survive the rapids."

We ride the rapids for over an hour. The sun is dipping toward the western horizon when we drag the kayak out of the river onto a sandy bend. We hang our drenched clothes on the surrounding bushes and don our few remaining dry clothes. In the twilight, we gather driftwood for a fire.

The fire crackles in the night. The river murmurs, chortles, hisses in the blackness. Stars dance overhead.

River Woman draws her knees to her chest and wraps her arms around them. Her eyes never leave the fire.

"You have much to learn," she says slowly. "And you have much to give."

I sink deeply into myself, aware of the fire, the stars, the river. I relax into a sense of kinship with each element of creation that surrounds me. The fire is alive. The river is alive. The stars are alive. I am alive.

"You did not come here to work," says the woman. Her voice surprises me, as her form had melded into fire and river in my awareness. "You are here to become."

Reflections by Vicki Noble

Vicki Noble is a feminist shamanic healer, author, scholar and wisdom teacher. After a profound awakening to the Goddess and Women's Spirituality in 1976, she collaborated with Karen Vogel to create the Motherpeace Tarot. She teaches in the Women's Spirituality programs at California Institute of Integral Studies and New College in San Francisco, sees private clients for astrology readings and healing sessions, and is working on the establishment of an ongoing training program for women in shamanic healing arts and Goddess spirituality. In her teaching she combines Buddhism, feminism, yoga, shamanism, and Goddess worship with a special focus on the female lineage of healers since ancient times. Vicki is the author of Motherpeace, Shakti Woman, Down is Up for Aaron Eagle, *and* Making Ritual with Motherpeace.

In a certain way, the Goddess tradition is a perfect preparation for menopause (or any other natural process in a woman's cycle) because the core of the tradition is cyclic time—birth, death, and rebirth. The art and artifacts from ancient cultures organized around a Goddess tend to observe, witness, and attempt to entrain with the natural cycles of life. Ancient lunar calendars are found as early as the Paleolithic period—notations on eagle bones and carved in stone, clocking the rhythmic timing of a woman's menstrual cycle or the number of months it takes a mare to carry a foal to term. Letting go into birth and death, acknowledging the changing of the seasons, the darkening of the Moon, the waxing and waning of all forms, nurtures acceptance and optimism in each of us, providing hope for the inevitable rebirth that follows any loss.

As menopause was approaching, and the transition that would be required was beginning to make itself known, I found it terribly difficult. I couldn't sleep, felt agitated and edgy most of the time (a friend described me as having a "short fuse"). I joked that I finally understood why so many women went on hormones! However, I was not interested in any chemical medicine myself, so I was determined to see it through in a natural way.

It was surprising to me (and disappointing) that my menopause turned out to be so hard. Because I had eaten organic food for twenty-some years, practiced daily yoga, and taken care of myself in such a focused way, I wrongly assumed my menopause would be a breeze. It was a nasty surprise when my hair thinned (even my precious, long eyelashes!), my face itched, and I had hot flashes every hour around the clock. I finally went to a

Chinese herbalist who gave me healing potions as well as hope, explaining that when the ovaries stop producing estrogen, it takes about a year and a half for the other organs to take up the slack. One must be patient and go with the flow, and eventually the body will come into its own new balance.

I was forced to correct almost everything in my life. I had to end a relationship that hadn't been working. I had to stop the busy travel schedule I had put in place for myself, in which I had been flying on airplanes at least once a month and more often during the summers. I could feel how the air travel upset my nervous system and put pressure on my kidneys, so I scaled down the travel for a couple of years to give my body a break. Drinking Chinese herbal tea saved my hair from falling out, but I still ended up having to cut my waist-long hair short as a response to the way the texture and tone had changed.

As a lifelong feminist, I was prepared to enjoy my aging process—determined to face the changes in my body and appearance with finesse. I knew there had to be a payoff in the transition, some kind of new power I would be able to access and channel after such a major life transition. I wasn't disappointed in this. The personal empowerment that comes with the ending of the menstrual periods is awesome. It was as if a switch had been flipped for me, a circuit reversed. The current of energy that had been my sexuality reversed itself and seemed to go up into my head, rather than down and out through my sexual expression. I was then able (willing) to realize for the first time in my life that I had literally been "driven" by the sexual energies that I had so enjoyed and cultivated ever since my adolescence.

All the time and energy that had gone into my relationships was suddenly freed up for creative endeavor. This has been a most welcome surprise for me. Even though I still spend loads of time with my son who lives at home and my grandchildren who live nearby, I am free to channel my creativity into projects, research, books, and spiritual practice—without the distraction and emotional upheaval that came with my intimate sexual relationships. I'm not saying this is necessarily the case for every woman, but for me it was a welcome change. I realized a deep truth one day in conversation with a friend when I said, "I've had enough good sex to last a lifetime!" When I heard myself say this, I realized how true it was, and I felt a tremendous joy and acceptance at being with myself rather than seeking a partner. It's as if I have waited my whole life to be lovers with myself and my work in this primary way, and now I am finally able to commit to it and not abandon myself. Whether this lasts the rest of my life or not, I have no idea—and I don't care. It's good enough for now.

I think one issue that is rarely mentioned is the pressure heterosexual women feel to remain attractive and sexually receptive to their male partners, even though their bodies are profoundly trying to change gears. The inner power that wants to be unleashed through the menopausal journey is a kind of high-functioning creativity and spiritual leadership that requires a different sexual rhythm than that of a younger woman. The fear (the threat) of a husband leaving a menopausal woman for a younger woman is all too real, and I think this plays into women's decisions to go on hormones and artificially extend their menstrual periods in order to "stay young" rather than making the biological transition and reaping the spiritual rewards. Ditto with all the cosmetic surgeries performed on menopausal women these days.

It seems to me that menopause forces an essential alignment within a woman, helping her to self-correct in terms of imbalances by simply making any excess impossible to sustain. The consequences are too unbearable and require that you change your behavior or your situation. (Of course, if you go to the doctor and take hormones, then you interfere with the natural process, putting it off for a later date and compounding your health problems.)

I would advise women to listen to their bodies for direction, taking the symptoms of the Change as cues. When my faced itched so badly I wanted to scratch it right off, I took up knitting and stayed home for three months instead of being socially active. When my hair fell out, I stopped flying so much. I even gave up spicy food for a while, a great sacrifice, and I took up eating oysters and yams at the suggestion of my acupuncturist. All of these various adaptations made a positive difference and eventually became part of my (new) regular patterns.

Spiritual practice and meditation are keys to survival during menopause. Without some form of calming the mind and soothing the agitation, I can't imagine being able to get through such a roller-coaster ride without hormones. I remember two occasions where my spiritual practices obviously made a physical difference in the symptoms of my menopause.

The first time was when I was in Oregon facilitating a "transformational healing ritual" in a public space for more than a hundred people. There was no drummer that day, so I picked up a drum and kept the steady beat for almost an hour, the required time for the ritual to be effective in terms of putting serious physical illnesses into remission. While the others present performed hands-on healing (usually my function), I drummed. When the ritual was over, my hourly hot flashes went away for more than a month.

The second time it happened was very similar, but this time I was in a Tibetan Buddhist retreat with Tsultrim Allione, from whom I learned my first Dakini practice. The first day of the retreat, Tsultrim and her community of experienced students performed the Chöd practice—a strong chanting practice that uses a drum and bell. Again my hot flashes disappeared for more than a month, letting me understand at a very deep level that they were energetically caused. From my experience, I would say that working with energy seems to be the most important treatment for the symptoms of menopause.

I don't know what anyone could have told me to prepare for menopause. I watched my own mother go through her menopause without hormones, bless her heart, and I knew it was doable. Indigenous women from other cultures don't seem to suffer the symptoms of menopause, so clearly the problem is related to Western lifestyle issues and choices. We spend our adult lives sitting in front of computers or at desks or whatever, and then when menopause comes along, the consequences catch up to us—our livers have to detox. Our processed diet; the pollution in the air, water, and food we take in; the speed and frenzy with which we approach our lives—all this matters, and it all comes up for redress during "the Change." Menopause has been pathologized in our culture, but it's a natural transition, a life phase—there's nothing wrong with it, and there's nothing wrong with women's bodies. The culprit is Western culture, and that's where we need to look for making changes if we want to regain a natural experience.

The other thing about it is that women in indigenous cultures are respected, even revered, after they stop bleeding. They become elders, sometimes shamans, and their tribes look to them for advice, guidance, and council. In our culture, we throw away older women, dismissing their experience as irrelevant, paying no heed to their wisdom and perceiving them as "uncool," which in our culture is a fate worse than death.

Vicki may be reached at: PO Box 1558, Freedom, CA 95019.
She can also be reached via her website, www@motherpeace.com, or by
e-mail: Vicki@motherpeace.com.

CHAPTER SIX

THE SCIENCE of TRANSFORMATION: EXTERNAL and INTERNAL LANDSCAPES

THE RIVER WE TRAVEL IS THE SAME, YET EACH ONE OF US IS UNIQUE IN HOW she will make the passage. The conditions will vary even on the same stretch of river on the same day, as our internal environment (thoughts, feelings, beliefs, and attitudes) has a profound effect on the outer environment (weather, climate, relationships, and so on) Will the river rise to flood stage? Will I have to carry the canoe over drought-parched sections of sandy river-bottom? Will wind howl, rain fly, or snow blanket the territory?

Personal strength also dictates the quality of the passage. Physical, mental, emotional, and spiritual stamina figure prominently in the outcome of the journey. We will discuss ways of developing these strengths. Endurance, how-ever, does not equal protection from the elements. Even the strongest, most capable woman may encounter conditions beyond her control or mastery. Those conditions may be external—a world war, an avalanche, a tsunami; the death of a parent, mate, or child. Personal inner changes may also demand attention, such as grief or diagnosis of a chronic or terminal illness.

EXTERNAL LANDSCAPES

During perimenopause, our external bodies change. Our hair begins to turn white or gray; wrinkles etch our faces. The body shape changes as estrogen and progesterone levels begin to drop (see chapter 3). Our physical "land-scape" begins to transform.

Simultaneously, the inner "body" or landscape also changes. We are shifting from one stage of the life journey to another. For some, the changes are matter of fact. For others, the transformation is so profound that the structure and contents of their former lives are completely obliterated.

Knowing that the journey will be unique for each woman, I offer the fol-lowing exploration of the landscapes you may traverse during this transi-tional time. These certainly are not the only templates; rather, they are meant to stretch the realm of possibility as you begin your travels, sketching your own map of your personal terrain of discovery. Rather than offering you lessons in geology, these landscapes are explorations in the science of transformation.

Many spiritual traditions have a deep understanding of the universe and our human role within that cosmological structure. In Tibetan Buddhist and Hu'na traditions, for example, our inner world is governed by the same principles that shape the outer world. In fact, our inner perceptions literally *create* the outer world.

After dissecting matter to its most fundamental units, quantum physicists are coming to the same conclusion: mind shapes matter. Our thoughts alter the external world. For so many generations, the Western scientific world has assumed that our mental development was influenced by the outer environment. "You are a product of your environment" has been the standard psychological cliché. Now we are discovering that influence is a two-way street: the environment influences the mind, and mind alters the environment.

The snake curls to bite its own tail. The scientific Western world, so entranced with dissecting matter into the smallest bits possible, turns inside out as those tiny particles lead scientists into the world of mysticism. The world of mystics, so long focused on the inner realms, suddenly finds common ground with physicists, mathematicians, and other scientists.

Kala H. Kos and John Selby in the book *The Power of Aloha* eloquently describe the convergence of inner and outer worlds, and the transformation that is possible when those worlds are united:

> . . .the Polynesian understanding of hu'na runs exactly parallel to the new scientific models of quantum reality in the field of wave mechanics, where two seemingly opposed principles or qualities (objective/subjective, cognitive/intuitive, male/female, doing/being, space/time, self/other, wave/particle, and so forth) exist only through their quality of being in complementary relationship to each other.
>
> Recently added to this list of complementary pairs in science (and known thousands of years ago in Hu'na) is what scientists now call the "consciousness/environment dialogue," where external reality continually and intimately influences internal consciousness, and vice versa.
>
> The key notion here regarding these linked pairs is that we can't have one without the other. As the Hu'na masters knew long ago, consciousness and the outer world are parts of a greater whole—

they're not distinct entities, as classic Cartesian science and our gen-
eral Western worldview have led us to believe.

The Hu'na tradition stands as one of the primary guides to har-
monizing our inner and outer experience purposefully so that,
instead of feeling we're victims of the outside world, we begin to
employ our conscious powers actively to influence the outer world
for our increased wellbeing and enjoyment.[1]

As noted earlier, menopause is not the only time women may experience
profound transformation. As one of the major gateways in the life cycle,
though, the potential for transformation is richly available. These
inner/outer landscapes offer examples of the many ways we can transition
from one stage of the life journey to another.

The Desert (Moving with Consciousness and Grounding)

Sparse. Clean. No extraneous elements clutter the desert. The earth demands
attentiveness in this place. All action must be accompanied by awareness in a
land where water is sparse. I cannot forget my water bottle or stumble at
midday hoping to find shelter from the desiccating rays of the sun.

I hike by myself across the open desert of Arches National Monument. I
have just finished a long course of study and am bone-hungry for solitude
and silence. I veer away from the well-traveled arches and find a quiet spot to
rest for the day. I crawl like a lizard under a bare-branched bush, sheltered
from the sweltering sun, and burrow into the red sand. I watch ants dragging
crumbs across the clean sand, diligent, oblivious of the heat. Golden sap
oozes from a broken branch, catching sunlight as cleanly as amber. Raven
caws into the stillness, the call reverberating off the nearby sandstone walls.
The call stands out like a meteor of sound in this silent landscape.

The desert demands consciousness matched with effective action. I am
respectful in this landscape. I do not walk with fear, but rather with silent
joy. Water is more useful than gold in this arid land, yet the landscape
quenches my soul in ways that no rainforest ever could. Space. Time. Open
mind. Sandy footprints. Peace.

Dr. Beth Davis, a naturopathic physician and gifted teacher of Native
American traditions, beautifully describes this state of balanced thought and
action in terms of brain function. "My main symptom (during menopause)
was my mind changing over from left to right brain, or maybe more balance

between the two hemispheres. That was a bit scary, but now I appreciate the more balanced perceptions."

The desert also encompasses choice, the ability to match conscious decision with action. Phyllis Rodin, a beloved elder now in her ninety-second year, recalls her choice to stop bleeding. "It was my fiftieth birthday, for goodness' sake, and that is certainly long enough for any woman to bleed. I decided that would be my last day of bleeding, and I've never bled since."

Ocean (Bliss, Moving with an Open Heart)

The sun is rising over the sand dunes to the east. I stand in the ocean, straining to see the farthest rim of the western horizon break with sprays of water as the dolphins head for shore. This is Monkey Mia, the west coast of Australia, where wild dolphins choose to interact with humans in knee-deep water. The desert air is still chilly this morning. I shiver in my damp bathing suit covered with a sweatshirt.

The sun strengthens. Dolphins weave gracefully through the water, pausing just before the sandy shore.

BB (Beautiful Baby) swims close to the humans already lining the shore. She carefully shields her baby, only about twenty-four-inches long, from human contact. The dolphins know that habituating the babies too early to humans can cause problems later.

I have spent two weeks with the dolphins, long enough to know their names and their dispositions. The researchers who have spent years at Monkey Mia say the dolphins require about as long to know us humans as we need to learn the dolphins' names. By that measure, I am sure the dolphins are intimately familiar with my body and some of my habits.

Today is my last day with the dolphins. My heart is full of love for these creatures. All of my movements are imbued with grace. Love extends throughout my whole body, filling my hands as I reach into the water to caress the passing dolphins. The dolphins have taught me this whole-body love, this bliss that blossoms far beyond my genitals. They have taught me to love unconditionally. Their love reaches across the barriers of land and sea, across species, and across the chasms of our minds and communications systems.

BB has made several passes in front of the humans now lining the shore. She and the baby swim toward me. Just inches before contact, BB slides her body behind me, so that the baby slides across my front.

Love explodes inside me, taking all thought with it. I am stunned by the touch of mother and baby, enveloping me in their maternal bond.

That moment rings in me, that moment of acceptance, acknowledgment—the best word I can offer is *blessing*. The dolphins, the ocean's finest ambassadors, teach me the territory of bliss, of openhearted joy. This is a love that goes beyond acceptance into full-being *embrace*.

In the words of Rumi, "There is so much magnificence, in the ocean. Waves are coming in, waves are coming in.. . ."[2] Those waves are bliss, moving in and through our being, moving us with a grace and wisdom beyond our land-locked comprehension.

The Abyss (Complete Disconnection from Self and Spirit)

Rain filters through the sodden beech trees, seeping into my parka as I move through them.. I circle this ancient Scottish hill as much to escape myself as the disappointment of the day. As the late afternoon glower deepens into evening, I am certain that if I fell off the face of the earth, no one would notice. I feel defeated, as if I have reached a roadblock on a dead-end road. I came here to grow, to stretch myself, to immerse myself in living a spiritual life. Instead of finding bliss, the community has become a highly polished mirror in which I must view myself, and I am dissatisfied with the reflection.

No, dissatisfied is not accurate. I am *horrified* by my own reflection. I have always thought of myself as a very self-aware person, but in this moment I feel completely severed from my soul and from Creator. Illness has plagued me for weeks. I have a persistent cough that I simply cannot shake. I long to escape the damp, cold, sea air of northern Scotland and flee to the Mediterranean, but even Italy lies blanketed with snow this winter. I am exhausted, and no amount of rest seems to replenish me.

I am dismayed at my inability to communicate with other people. Every statement seems to twist in my mouth and emerge crippled from my lips, the meaning mangled in the delivery. I am not sure how much of the "miscommunication" is mine, and how much belongs to others. I am certain that if I could only learn to love unconditionally, my words would ring true. I am sure that if I could clearly hear Creator's guidance, I would be healed. If only I could "learn my lessons," I would bridge this chasm that separates me from Creator.

Gradually I realize I have entered the abyss, a place of complete and total separation. Much like Persephone's journey, I am moving deeply into the underworld of my own soul. On this journey, I will discard all that no longer serves me: self-doubt, defunct relationships, assumptions engrained by my family upbringing. I will "die" to the old and make way for the new.

Many spiritual traditions refer to this transformation as "the dark night of the soul." One model that has helped me grasp this transformation is based on a twelve-hour clock. A complete circuit represents full spiritual evolution.

From noon to 3 P.M., the primary focus is on personal survival. Even if someone is deeply spiritual or religious, her primary concern at this turn of the clock is personal survival.

From 3 to 6 P.M. the primary focus is group survival. Many great business and community leaders inhabit this segment of the clock.

6 P.M. marks "the dark night of the soul." Crossing this line represents an enormous evolutionary shift. From this point onward, the primary focus is on what goes on *behind* the eyes rather than in front of them. The inner landscape is more compelling than the outer. Service becomes more and more important from 6 P.M. onward.

Many people deeply struggle during this transition. They grind back and forth over that 6 P.M. mark, not ready to move forward and reluctant to move back. I once asked a Lutheran pastor if he recognized this passage in his own tradition. "Of course," he commented. "That's what those Old Testament prophets were doing, wandering around in the desert for forty years."

I hope your own transition will be quicker and easier than Elijah's. I know from my own experience that the abyss, or dark night of the soul, was difficult on all levels. I suffered with chronic-fatigue-like symptoms. I simply could not regain my energy. I took three days away from the Findhorn Foundation, the community where I was living, to recover. Within a day of my return, I was exhausted again. About a month later, I spent a week with a friend of the community, a wise and salty elder named John. His Cockney-London humor and understated healing ways helped me finally begin my ascent from the abyss.

One analogy for understanding this passage is shifting from 120 volts of electricity to running 500 or 1000 volts of energy. For many, illness accompanies the transition simply because of the profound recalibration the body must endure.

Passing the 6 P.M. mark does not excuse anyone from paying the bills or taking the children to dental appointments. I still have to "take care of business" on the physical level. From that point onward, however, my inner world was more compelling than outer events.

9 P.M. on the clock represents full awakening. "Enlightenment" is a byproduct of that awakening. From 9 P.M. onward, the primary focus is on service. Gradually over the years I have learned that many famous (pop) spiritual leaders have never entered this segment of the clock. Jesus, Mohammed, and Buddha dwelled chiefly in this realm. Many "ordinary," unrecognized people also inhabit this sector. They are quietly focused on serving humanity and all of creation.

Beyond 10:00 or 10:30 P.M., most beings can no longer maintain a physical form. They move into the realm of pure spirit.

Bliss moves us like a rainbow arc from one state of being to another. In contrast, the abyss moves us *at depth* into a new way of being.

Mountaintop (Personal Transformation)

The climb is long, my pack heavy. The sun stalls overhead in the pristine blue Wyoming sky. Sweat erupts under my pack, then dries into a salty crust when I stop to rest. The last scramble to the summit traverses a scree slope, with rocks and pebbles giving way beneath my hiking boots.

Three days of backpacking preceded this summit climb. We left heavier packs at last night's campsite to make this ascent. The days of driving, the strain of heavy packs, and the challenge of unfamiliar territory culminate in this moment as I finally place my foot on the summit.

From this height, I can see ten snow-covered peaks. I can look over the vast territory that surrounds us and mentally sketch the trail that led us to this place. That arduous trail appears as a dollhouse miniature, a footnote in this vast landscape. As I rest on the summit, I can clearly see the journey that has led me to this place. That journey includes inner navigation as well as physical movement. I view the choices that have led me to this vista, and know myself better for that reflection.

Our guide is gesturing to the south, pointing out the valleys and lakes we will traverse on our three-day descent. From this height I have a magnificent sense of expansion and ease, viewing the territory ahead. I have accomplished what I thought was impossible; the descent, no matter how challenging, is a denouement in comparison.

This enlarged view also gives me an opportunity to expand my view of life. I cut the restraints of my usual conditioned thinking; I drop my list of assumptions along with my pack. Here I am free to expand, to dream, and to reconstruct the territory of my mind. This peak is more than a mountain; this peak is a heightened understanding of myself and my place in the world. This view is as much internal as external.

Deep breath. Relaxation after a long struggle. Accomplishment. Rest before the descent. Yes, eventually I must return to the world, to my daily routine. I will return, however, with a new landscape within me, an expanded view of where I have been and where I am heading. I have been to the mountaintop, and the journey has expanded me and allowed me to reshape my inner territory.

The Volcano (Planetary Transformation)

Walking to the edge of the Haleakala Crater on the island of Maui, I look down into a primordial world, the land freshly made from the bowels of the earth. This island is the aftermath of volcanic eruptions that pushed from the ocean floor to the surface, and then rose another ten thousand feet. Swathes of reds, greens, and golds sweep across the volcanic cones jutting in the caldera, as if Pele herself had spontaneously flung her paint pot on these dramatic slopes. The landscape is elemental—rock, sky, cloud. The features are as primordial as any dinosaur fantasy I have ever nurtured. This is truly a place shaped by profound, elemental forces.

After three days of backpacking and fasting, my body slows to a reptilian pace. I am nearing the Halalii cone, where the last lava spouted two hundred years ago. The core of that vent plummets sixty-five feet into the earth.

I sit down to drink water. My hunger-dulled mind takes in the landscape without comment. I try to eat a few bites of dried fruit to bolster me. Even this tiny amount of food churns in my stomach. Wracked with nausea, I stumble to the edge of the vent and look down into the darkness.

I plod onward another three miles to the campsite. I put up my tent. Looking around me, I cannot recall where I am. I sit down inside the tent and close my eyes. I am the elements. Nothing more, nothing less. Like the cones around me, I am rock, I am molten fire, I am water, I am sky.

The volcano has stripped me to bare elements. I don't even have the template of "me" to reshape those elements. I am raw, pushing upward, nameless, placeless. I am the first, unedited expression of landscape. In time, I sense the rain and wind will shape me into some form, but for now I embody the primordial power of the elements.

A volcanic eruption affects much more than the mountain peak or even the surrounding countryside. Lava erupts and reshapes the surrounding landscape, but the winds of change carry the ash for thousands of miles. The earth renews itself during these vast eruptions, bringing the molten core of the earth upward and outward to form new land at the surface. The volcanic ash renews the soil, distributing much needed nutrients over vast territories.

The volcano has the power to transform itself as well as everything around it.

For some women, menopause can transform their lives with the same power and force as a volcano. She may be radically different in how she lives and moves in the world, and this transformation affects all those around her. Living in the midst of the volcano, that deep, profound change may not be so obvious to the individual woman. The transformation is simply part of her daily landscape, just as the eruption was simply part of the geological schedule for Haleakala. Sometimes the change is more obvious to those living and working with her.

One of the women who comes to mind when I think of volcanic change is Rachel Carson. Both a gifted writer and a scientist, she used her knowledge and skill to alert the world to the dangers of pesticides and insecticides. After her book The Edge of the Sea was published, people began to send her studies about the effects of pesticides on the land, water, and wildlife that surround us. A deeply devoted scientist, she wanted definitive documentation to confirm the effects of pesticides. She combined the rigor of scientific study with the eloquence of her writing. That combination of art and science reached people in ways that facts alone never could. Her passion, combined with scientific rigor, catalyzed first awareness and then profound change in the way we use pesticides.

Rachel wrote Silent Spring, her final book, knowing she was dying of breast cancer. She did not "go gently into that night;" she went out burning with a sense of mission. She was only fifty-six when she died, yet she left a body of work that continues to challenge and inspire us.

Caterpillar to Chrysalis

Perimenopause marks the inward turning of the caterpillar, weaving its cocoon in preparation for transformation. For some, the journey will be matter-of-fact, like the consciously grounded passage across a desert landscape. For others, the changes will be profound, like volcanic lava rushing from the earth's core to create new forms. Each passage brings its own wisdom, its own gifts and challenges. May your journey be blessed, no matter what landscape(s) you traverse.

MAPPING YOUR INNER LANDSCAPE

Sometimes the terrain of our inner journey is not obvious until we look back on the landscape. Our conscious mind rarely knows where we are headed. Our dreams and meditations, though, portals to the deeper, wilder, wiser mind, often have both compass and map to point the way.

I offer the following exercises to befriend the landscape you are traversing, and draw upon the "wild mind" for reconnaissance/guidance on your journey.

EXERCISES

- Acquaint yourself with your "dream keeper." Many native traditions understand that a wise aspect of ourselves stewards our dreams. You can call upon this dream keeper to guide your nocturnal wanderings so that you can gather the wisdom, healing, or insight you need and bring it back to your waking world. Before falling asleep, set your intention. Most nights, I ask that my dreams support my spiritual evolution. I also request that I may be able to bring the wisdom and insight I need back into my waking consciousness.

- Keep a journal close to your bed. When you have revelatory dreams, you will want a place to record them. You may also choose to have a small tape recorder by your bed to record your dreams. You can train yourself to remember dreams. I often hold on to a shred of a dream, like clinging to the edge of a robe. As I begin to record a dream, other sections of dream often come back to me. Train yourself to retain a few details of the dream, and you will soon be able to able to draw the entire dream through the veil.

- Plant the seed of a question before going to sleep. Ask for assistance if you need it. One night Judith Pintar asked her dream keeper for guidance about sharing her knowledge of Ojibway/Anishnabe sacred traditions. In the morning, she discovered she had written the entire outline for a set of divination cards based on the Ojibway teachings of the seven directions. She had no memory of waking during the night. Thankfully her journal was there to capture the ephemeral whisperings of her dreams. *A Voice from the Earth: The Cards of Winds and Changes* is Judith's fulfillment of her dream.[3]

♦ In meditation, ask to move through your sacred inner landscape. Be open to unexpected adventures and unfamiliar territories. You may have a sense of "layers" within your being. Some might conceive of these layers as "chakras," but the sacred terrain I'm addressing is actually much deeper, much closer to the soul level. The chakras have more to do with our physical interface with spirit. The landscapes I'm addressing here have more to do with the soul's terrain. In my first meditative journey to explore this territory, I was surprised to enter a brown-sand desert. I wondered if the territory reflected an emotionally barren life. As I settled into the desert, though, I experienced a deeply nourishing peace. I realized I have been drawn to several desert regions in my outer life, all of which have profoundly influenced my inner world. I crave silence and open space, both of which are plentiful in the desert. I also moved through a lush forest environment and on to other territories. Take notes. Make the journey several times. Allow yourself to be surprised by what you find.

Reflections by Patricia Willer

Patricia Weller has been an artist and teacher for thirty-five years. On a lifelong quest to unpeel her own onion, she has enjoyed many careers including mother, therapist, art teacher, counselor, organic farmer, and herbalist, to name a few. She leaped (sans parachute) into creating full-time twenty years ago. Soon realizing that some of her work had an empowering nature for others, she concentrated on embellishments that act also as talismans not only to delight but also to inspire, remind, and assist us in our journey of body and spirit. Her "Goddesses with an Attitude" have become her specialty.

The Roman Catholic tradition I was raised in did not include the word "menopause." Nor can I recall the word ever being mentioned in my home as I was growing up. I have had to create my own spiritual traditions, and fortunately that has involved exposure to some very fine wise women. I noticed the abundance of creative woman who only began their creative journey in their fifties or later. That gave me a positive future to look toward, but I don't believe I attributed that to menopause until I personally experienced it.

Because I knew next to nothing about menopause, I didn't have the expectation that I would be endlessly depressed, lose my sexuality, or dry up, which are some of the beliefs I have noted in friends. It may be entirely a projection on my part, but it seemed that those woman whose primary self-worth was involved with either being a mother or having a man's love had a more difficult menopause. Wow, that sounds really uppity, doesn't it? Still, with few exceptions, it seems to hold true in my personal experience.

I also believe that my experience with menopause, so positive in comparison, was affected by the fact that I was developing a new and very creative career. There were great risks, battles with fear, and leaps of faith, but also great rewards to my self-esteem. It seems a bit murkier looking back as I write this. I assumed the career change helped the menopause, but now I question whether perhaps the menopause was a great motivator for the career change. I also wonder if menopause amplified some of the absolute exhaustion and fear I experienced while starting my business.

I delight that sharing this brings out new realms for me to ponder.

I was very young, in my mid-forties, when I went into menopause. I was working as director of a teen center, which was quite challenging, and had recently gotten remarried, to a man with four children. I had my first hot flash in a cave, or perhaps it was the temperature of the cave that made me "own the experience" as a hot flash. The hot flashes continued, and my sleep was quite disrupted over a period of about six months. I vividly recall driving down my driveway one day. When I began the journey of perhaps 250 yards, all was right with my world. By the end of that brief journey, I wanted to kill! The transition was so obvious and unexpected, denial was impossible, and I recall thinking, "Aha! This is menopause!"

In my recollection (ah, hindsight!), hot flashes caused the most discomfort. My marriage was not a good one, and the children—almost grown but completely untrained—were a huge challenge. I have often thought that George married me primarily so that I could prepare his children for the world before they went out and did serious damage. Still, with the help of my amazing son Forrest who was then in high school, those kids came around and actually seemed happy and productive. Although that period was difficult, my focus, direction, and energy were quite good.

One morning after a long night of hot flashes I realized I was letting this thing control me and that I needed to take action. I did two things. First, I began using self-hypnosis for the hot flashes. This is a tool I have long used with great success for pain and many other needs. I had not been using it recently but recalled that I had often used it to bring about minor temperature changes. If I was chilly or enduring uncomfortable heat, I would use hypnosis to release the discomfort. At the first sign of a hot flash, and fortunately you do get a warning, I would use my hypnosis to stabilize my body temperature. I also wrote affirmations for myself that reinforced my body making these changes with ease and grace, which I repeated daily using deep hypnosis.

Second, I gathered what information I could about menopause, which is when I realized there was very little real information out there. Some of what had been written, mostly by male doctors, was indeed humorous, and most sources were in complete contradiction with each other. I began with Germaine Greer's book and followed up with several books written by American Indian wise women. Unfortunately I passed these books on to others in need and have no recollection of authors' names (other than Greer's) or titles.

The most important information I found was a collection of herbs used by the wise women of old, from earth-based, natural cultures. Armed with my list, I went to a health-food store prepared to create my own concoction. I was blessed in that the woman who helped me had recently done similar research. She pointed out several ready-made products that included all the herbs on my list. The one I chose was "Change of Life." Another friend supplied me with a homeopathic concoction called "Menopause." They were tiny pills intended to wake the body to produce its own variation of the needed cure.

Over the next six months, the combination of hypnosis and herbs gradually faded all ill effects. Most symptoms were gone within three months, but I continued the herbs for six.

What do I wish someone had told me about menopause, and what do I wish to share? That is the most important question, because I was completely surprised by the liberating, empowering effects of making the menopausal transition. I hope I can convey this properly, because there is so much emphasis on the misery of the process and none on the positive effects of the transition.

During the different sections of a woman's life—maiden, mother and crone—we have dramatically different needs, physically and emotionally. I believe that our bodies do a fantastic job of producing what we need. The energies that are first directed toward learning and developing (maiden)and then toward sexual attraction, nurturing, productivity, and endurance (mother), do not die or shrivel up. After menopause, those energies are at our disposal to redirect in any way we choose. In some ways, this is actually easier because they are no longer so tied to the hormonal roller coaster.

The delightful surprise of menopause was the release of much that was hormonally driven. I used to think I had done some very stupid things during my life. Now I am able to look back and see how many of those things were driven in large part by hormones. Although I considered myself very liberated, I can see how my need to partner overruled rational thought. I also see how my need to protect my children at times caused me not to direct them as well as I might have. These are just two examples.

I have attempted to learn, grow, and improve during this life, and by this point I do feel that all that effort and all those "learning experiences" have served to create a better person. Call it mellowed, attained wisdom, whatever, my perspective seems more in balance and harmony. I have realized the huge toll that emotional upheaval causes me, and so I find no use for the drama queen I used so well at age twenty. I seem far more able to release judgment of myself and others. I *know* I can't do it all, and finally feel fine about that. These are just a few of the things I'm grateful for in my experience of cronehood. These joys cannot be attributed to menopause, effort, or intention alone, but all these things seemed to come together and jell after the transition and release of menopause.

I have found a wonderful community of elder woman, and together we are facing the interesting changes and trials of growing older. I can't shout loudly enough about how empowering support is during this time of life. I have tried to deal with major changes alone, and I have learned the power of sharing and having supportive community. The difference is vast and I'm sure it has much impact on how we cope.

There was a time around six years ago when I was doing much caregiving for my mother. Although we are very different mentally and emotionally, we are very similar physically. She has resisted aging and resented the loss of the two things that were her priorities in this life: physical beauty and career. She has been unable or unwilling to transfer those passions to other productive activities. Never having interest in hobbies, literature, or exercise, the inevitable loss of her only interests left her bitter and resentful. She simply stopped learning or attempting anything new, and thus began a steady decline both mentally and physically.

It took a long while for me to realize I could not save her, and during that time I allowed some of her very limited perspective to leak into my consciousness. I began to have a fearful view of my future and aging.

I was saved from this by attending my first Crones Counsel. Crones Counsel is an organization whose mission is to honor elder women's wisdom and accomplishments.

At my first counsel, we honored seventeen women over eighty years old, and I wondered at their beauty and vitality. These woman and the many others entering or experiencing cronehood had not lost interest in life. They remained involved and continued to learn and, more importantly, to share or teach what life had taught them.

I am embarrassed to admit that the thought of honoring my elders had never really occurred to me, as I was too busy avoiding what they were to ever consider what they had endured, created, transformed. Only when I was able to really accept my female ancestors for all that they did achieve, especially considering what they were taught, was I able to release any resentments and begin to cherish them. The women at Crones Counsel presented me with an alternate reality for aging. With the support of these amazing women, I released much of the negative, suffering beliefs that our society often associates with aging and was able to create a blueprint for living this last portion of my life to its fullest. I am realizing now that on the journey to become the best that I can be, I have perhaps only just begun the most exciting part.

Patricia Weller can be reached at druidwoman@aol.com or: PO Box 595, 316 Box Elder Avenue, Paonia, CO 81428; (970) 527-5421; (970) 596-1118

For information about Crones Counsel, visit: www.cronescounsel.net

CHAPTER SEVEN

OUR CHANGING BODIES: HORMONAL and CYCLICAL CHANGE

Earlier we introduced menopause, perimenopause, and reproductive years. To refresh everyone's memory, I'll briefly define each of those before we move into a deeper exploration of our changing bodies.

STAGES IN A WOMAN'S LIFE CYCLE

Menopause officially begins after one full year with no menstrual bleeding. You may enter menopause as early as your late twenties or as late as your sixties. By medical definition, women who begin menopause before age forty have an "early menopause." The average age in North America is fifty-one years.

Peri means "around," so ***perimenopause*** means "around the time of menopause." This transitional period may last from six months to ten years. If the average North American woman enters menopause at fifty-one years old, she may have begun noticing changes (for example, mild hot flashes, menstrual cycle irregularities, and so on) as early as age forty or forty-one.

During her **reproductive years**, a woman ovulates, menstruates, and has the potential to become pregnant.

We will explore these stages in chronological order, beginning with reproductive years.

Reproductive Years

Your menstrual cycle begins with the first day of bleeding. A full cycle lasts from the first day of menstrual bleeding until the next first day of bleeding. Often when asked the length of her menstrual cycle, a woman will say, "Oh, five or six days." She is telling me about her bleeding, the first few days of the cycle, but not the entire cycle.

During this first part of the cycle, both estrogen and progesterone levels are very low, which is why most women do not take reproductive hormones while bleeding. When your uterus finishes shedding the lining, estrogen levels begin to rise. Remember that estrogen stimulates growth. The endometrium begins to thicken, and follicles in the ovary grow. The follicles are like tiny balloons with eggs inside. During your reproductive years, the ovary contains follicles in all different stages of development. Some are barely developed while others are close to maturation. The rise in estrogen signals the follicles to continue developing.

Near the time of ovulation, the ovary singles out one follicle that is almost fully mature. Several hormones surge to encourage this balloonlike follicle to burst and release the egg. Progesterone rises slightly just before ovulation and estrogens spike, reaching their highest peak in the cycle. The pituitary gland makes two hormones that also catalyze the follicle to open: follicle stimulating hormone (FSH) and leutenizing hormone (LH). Ovulation occurs at the moment the follicle bursts. The freed ovum then makes its way to the uterine (or "fallopian") tube where it begins its journey to the uterus.

Occasionally more than one follicle fully matures and releases an egg. Clomid and other fertility drugs encourage multiple follicles to ovulate, which explains the higher incidence of multiple births with fertility drugs. During perimenopause, the ovaries lose follicles at a higher rate,[1] which may account for why women in their forties are more likely to give birth to fraternal (non-identical) twins. Elevated FSH and decreased inhibin levels (see below) could account for this trend. Usually, however, only one follicle fully matures.

Ovulation lasts for only a brief moment. Although many women have no sensation, some experience a "pinch" or cramp in their lower abdomen at the time of ovulation. *Mittelschmerz*, a German word meaning "pain in the middle," referring to midcycle pain, is the medical term for this sensation. You may also feel heaviness or cramping that can last several hours, or even a day or two.

After releasing the egg, the follicle transforms into the "corpus luteum" and starts making progesterone. LH, produced by the pituitary gland, promotes this transformation. Libido rises along with progesterone levels, precisely when you are fertile. Progesterone also signals the uterus to hold onto the endometrium, which is vital in maintaining a pregnancy if the ovum is fertilized. If the corpus luteum does not produce enough progesterone, the uterus cannot maintain the lining, and the endometrium sloughs off, aborting the fetus.

After ovulation, the corpus luteum produces 20 to 30 mg of progesterone a day. If the ovum is fertilized, progesterone continues to rise throughout pregnancy, reaching 300 to 600 mg per day by the end of the third trimester. If the ovum is not fertilized, however, progesterone and estrogen levels drop, and the endometrium begins to shed. Your "period" begins, with the first day of bleeding marking the beginning of a new cycle.

The average time from ovulation to the onset of bleeding (the "luteal phase") is fourteen days. The time can vary from ten to eighteen days, but on average the luteal phase lasts fourteen days. The timing is usually consistent for each woman. A woman with a fourteen-day luteal phase, for example, almost always ovulates fourteen days before she begins bleeding. This last phase of the menstrual cycle is the predictable part of the cycle. The follicular phase (from the onset of bleeding to ovulation) may vary, but the luteal phase remains constant.

Perimenopause

Some women groan when they hear perimenopause can last from six months to ten years: "Ten years! I'll never make it!" This seemingly long transition time, however, is a blessing in disguise because the body has time to adjust to the hormonal changes. Perimenopause officially begins with the first noticeable symptoms, which are unique to each woman. Some women may experience an occasional hot flash, others may notice a change in their menstrual bleeding, many have more pronounced PMS symptoms, and still others have no symptoms whatsoever.

Estrogen levels fluctuate during perimenopause, finally stabilizing by the end of menopause at about 40 to 60 percent of the amount produced during reproductive years. Progesterone, however, drops to almost nothing, even before the end of perimenopause. Let's look at the menstrual cycle to understand what causes this drop in progesterone.

As you approach menopause, estrogens continue to cycle. You build the endometrium as estrogen levels rise and then at least partially shed the uterine lining when estrogens drop. During perimenopause, however, you may stop ovulating, even though you continue to have periods.

Most of us assume we must be ovulating if we have a period. Not necessarily so, particularly as we near menopause. Something similar happens in early adolescence: the ovaries sporadically ovulate before finally developing a regular rhythm. The same pattern repeats itself in late perimenopause. The ovaries may cough and sputter, occasionally skipping an ovulation, until the last year or two before menopause when a woman may not ovulate at all.

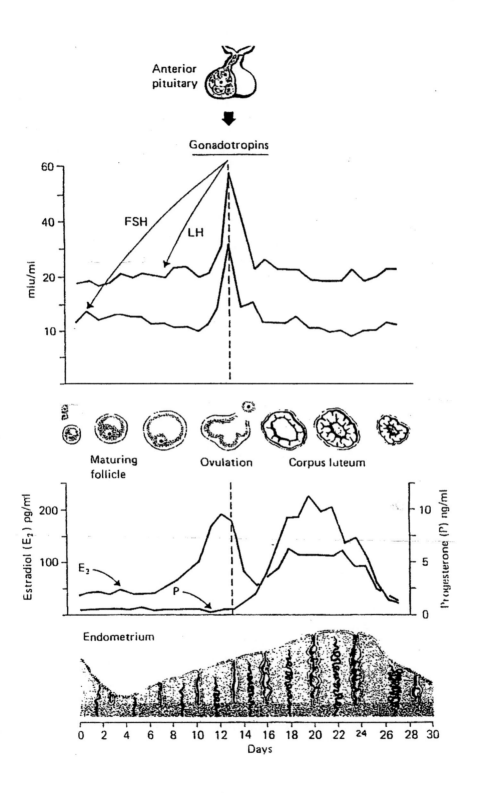

If you do not ovulate, you do not make a corpus luteum, and therefore your ovary produces no progesterone. The ovary must ovulate before it can produce progesterone. The adrenal gland makes a small backup supply of progesterone but falls far short of the amount the ovary would normally produce.

When a woman stops ovulating and progesterone levels drop, she suddenly has relatively more estrogen activity. With very little progesterone to balance, she has a tendency to develop what are called "estrogen dominance" symptoms. Look at the list of estrogens' functions in chapter 3 and consider what those normal tendencies would look like in excess.

ESTROGEN DOMINANCE SYMPTOMS

- ◆ Heavy menstrual bleeding, due to overgrowth of the endometrium, because the ovary produces no progesterone to slow the growth of the uterine lining.

- ◆ Increased blood-sugar levels. Initially the body may overreact to elevated blood-sugar levels by producing too much insulin, causing blood-sugar levels to plummet. When blood sugar is low, food cravings develop, particularly for sugar or simple carbohydrates such as pastries, chocolate, and pasta. A woman eats these foods, her blood sugar skyrockets momentarily and then comes crashing down, and the cravings start all over again.

- ◆ Mood swings, which often fluctuate in tandem with blood sugar.

- ◆ Water retention, bloating, swelling. Increased water retention may also lead to high blood pressure.

- ◆ Irritability, nervousness, anxiety, due to overstimulation of the nervous system.

- ◆ Increased fat deposition, particularly in breasts and hips.

- ◆ Decreased libido, due to lower progesterone levels.

- ◆ Breast soreness and tenderness. Estrogen stimulates breast cells to divide quickly without fully maturing.

In earlier years, we would call these symptoms PMS. Many perimenopausal women, some of whom have never experienced PMS, report developing raging premenstrual symptoms as they approach menopause.

Long-term Estrogen Dominance

Long-term estrogen dominance may also lead to more pronounced symptoms:

- Fibrocystic breasts or breast cancer. Women with fibrocystic breast syndrome do *not* have increased risk of developing breast cancer. Increased estrogen, however, can cause or exacerbate both conditions.

- Uterine fibroids. Estrogen stimulates growth of the uterus, and uterine fibroids are a benign overgrowth of the uterus. Fibroids become problematic if they cause excessive menstrual bleeding or begin to press on other structures such as the bladder, spine, or intestines.

- Endometriosis, which develops when endometrial tissue migrates outside the uterus, for example, to the abdominal wall or ovaries. This tissue grows in response to estrogen but cannot shed like a normal lining in the uterus. Instead, the areas scar, sometimes causing tremendous pain. Eventually the scarring may cause damage as well, for example, creating adhesions on the intestines.

Obviously younger women may also develop these conditions, but the tendency for estrogen dominance explains why perimenopausal women are more prone to develop endometriosis, fibrocystic breasts, and/or uterine fibroids as they near menopause. These three conditions often develop in the same woman, again pointing to the common instigator—estrogen, a growth-related hormone, that can cause overgrowth in excessive amounts.

FSH, LH, AND PERIMENOPAUSE

Normally FSH and LH surge at the time of ovulation. When a perimenopausal woman does not ovulate, her pituitary gland notices the ovary did not release an egg. "What do you mean, you're not ovulating?" says the pituitary gland to the ovary. "You've always ovulated at this time." The pituitary gland proceeds to make more and more FSH and LH, trying to flog the ovary into ovulating.

"I'm tired," says the ovary. "Don't bother me." The ovary does not release an egg.

Your doctor may order FSH and/or LH blood tests to determine whether you are perimenopausal. Elevated FSH and LH levels usually mean the pituitary gland is desperately signaling the exhausted ovary to release an egg. These two hormones normally rise at the time of ovulation, so the best time to test FSH and LH would be at your usual ovulation time, which is usually fourteen days before your period is due. If your periods are erratic, testing FSH and LH becomes a crap shoot. You may not know exactly when or if you are ovulating. A blood draw several days before or after ovulation may miss the spike in FSH and LH. Remember, too, you may ovulate sporadically as you near menopause. If the test is done during an ovulatory month, FSH and LH levels will be normal. The test may show elevated FSH levels one month and normal levels the next.

The point here is that FSH and LH tests cannot predict with 100 percent accuracy whether or not you are perimenopausal. In addition, the transition through perimenopause is not always a steady one. Trauma may accelerate your journey through perimenopause; conversely, resolving stress can slow or temporarily reverse the passage. One woman, for example, began to have severe hot flashes shortly after her husband's death. Lab tests showed elevated FSH levels, and the physician assumed she was well into perimenopause. A year later, however, after a period of grieving and reevaluation, the hot flashes stopped, her periods became regular, and FSH levels dropped to normal. Grief moved her closer to menopause, and resolution of the stress reversed the progression. Of course she will eventually move toward menopause again, and the hot flashes may return. The passage through perimenopause is not always a steady, predictable progression of events.

During perimenopause, elevated FSH levels stimulate increased estrogen production. Contrary to the popular notion that estrogen production drops during perimenopause, we have evidence that many women's estrogen levels actually increase.[2, 3, 4]

In postmenopausal women, FSH and LH levels return to normal. The pituitary gland finally gets the message that the ovaries are in permanent retirement and stops trying to flog the ovaries into ovulating.

Menopause

Some women ask if menopause begins when the ovaries run out of eggs. Actually we never use all our eggs. The ovaries, including all of our eggs, develop by the time we are a four-month-old fetus. At birth, our ovaries house approximately 250,000 follicles. Fortunately we never have 250,000 menstrual periods! We enter menopause not when we run out of eggs, but rather when the ovary reaches the end of its reproductive cycle. The body reabsorbs the thousands of remaining follicles in the ovary.

Certain events can speed our entry into menopause. We have already discussed how trauma (physical and emotional) can hasten the transition into menopause. Chemically induced menopause (for example, chemotherapy) can occur in a matter of months. Some women's ovaries return to normal after chemotherapy, others' ovaries do not. Oophorectomy, surgical removal of the ovaries, catapults a woman into menopause within twenty-four hours. Without the luxury of a six-month to ten-year adjustment period, she may experience harsher, more prolonged symptoms than a woman who transitions naturally through perimenopause.

After menopause, hormone levels remain fairly stable. Estrogen levels are about 40 to 60 percent of what they were during reproductive years, while progesterone plummets to almost nothing. Testosterone levels remain relatively unchanged, unless a woman has an oophorectomy, in which case testosterone levels drop by about one-half.

These postmenopausal hormone levels are normal, natural changes. Some elderly women remain healthy with no hormone supplementation while others may require hormone replacement therapy. No two women make the passage into their elder years the same way; therefore, each woman is unique in the supplements she will or will not need after menopause. In chapter 8, we will explore the symptoms and risk factors that provide clues to whether or not a woman may need hormone replacement therapy.

SEX AND CREATIVITY

For many women, menopause changes both body image and sexuality. For some, menopause increases libido, as the ongoing worry about pregnancy passes. For others, sexual appetite plummets as creative (and sometimes physical) energy is diverted elsewhere in their lives.

In meditation one day, I asked River Woman for her insights about sex, sexuality, and creativity during the menopause. Knowing the diversity of women's experience, I was eager for her wisdom:

"River Woman, speak to me of sex."

She laughs, her head tipped back, the sounds erupting from deep in her belly.

"Sex is much bigger than physically mingling with one person. Sex is about *intimacy*, with earth, with cosmos. I have sex by merging my essence with the soul or presence of another being. Sex is so much more than physical contact.

"The intimacy is with life itself. Remember, you are preparing to shed this physical envelope, like a cicada discarding its translucent shell.

"The physical body is still important, but your mind and soul predominate now. You have more mastery of the physical vehicle as it slows. Of course the body is still important. Right relationship with this physical earth, this orbit of life, bonds you more deeply with the source of life.

"The physical body truly becomes a vehicle when you are in right relationship. The body is a source of pleasure and deep connection—with the land, with another's soul, with creation.

"You will also develop, simultaneously, more detachment. Ah, yes, this is my body, *my* body, not a disconnected *'the'* body. This is *my* body, *and* I have other equally important aspects of myself. Thus, when the body begins to wear, like a ship gradually breaking apart at the edges of the sea, you are aware but not distraught. You have a body, but you are not your body. Your soul inhabits the physical vehicle rather than the body wooing the soul."

River Woman pauses, drawing a deep breath. "That may not be accurate. The body and soul are constantly wooing one another. Let's say the arrangement becomes more matter-of-fact, less hormonally driven, just as we fuel our personal relationships differently.

"Hormones are no longer the currency. Love, relevance, grace, insight become the primary fuels. Do you understand?"

Reluctantly I nod. I wonder if I have squandered my hotly charged, hormonally driven years. I think back to my twenties and how I wish I had had the financial savvy to deposit my small savings into an IRA. I wasn't using the money at the time, and I had no understanding of compounding interest.

I wonder if I've also missed making relationship investments. I realized with some regret at my parents' fiftieth wedding anniversary party that I would never celebrate a similar event until my mid-nineties, if at all.

Was I squandering my last few years of relatively youthful appearance, before all of my golden hair was exchanged for silver, by not searching for a mate? Would I regret in my sixties that I had not invested in relationship now?

River Woman joins me at the beach. I know she has an uncanny ability to read my thoughts. We watch waves grinding stones, shells, glass, and plastic with their churning movements.

"Nothing withstands the waves," comments River Woman. "You came in alone, and you will exit alone. Your financial and relationship portfolios won't survive the sea's action."

"If nothing matters, how can I know how best to direct my life?"

River Woman smiles slowly.

"Nothing matters, and everything matters. Take your choice. Both are true."

"So I possess a dangerous freedom, don't I?"

"Dangerous?" She looks puzzled. "Why dangerous?"

"I'm free from right or wrong, the correct or incorrect course of action. I can't rely on anything outside myself to direct my choices."

River Woman's face brightens. "Yes, you got it there at the end. Only you can direct and organize the elements. Fashion them to your liking. Just know that natural forces will eventually return them to their purest form. You can't be attached to their forms, because they are always changing— building up, washing away, building up again. Enjoy the scenery. It doesn't last long."

Love, Lovers, and the Creative Muse

Many peri- and menopausal women seek help for reduced libido. I always ask, "Is that a problem for you, or for your partner?"

Most report the problem rests with their partner. "And I suppose it's a problem for me, too, because I want to have a good relationship. I'm just not interested anymore. Is there something wrong with me?"

My sense from conversations with many women is that instead of "drying up" sexually, they begin to divert sexual energy into other forms of creativity. Vicki Noble eloquently describes taking herself seriously as her own lover, and directing sexual energy into her creative projects.

"I just don't *think* about sex," many women report. "It's just not part of my consciousness anymore."

Of course each woman is different, and some feel much freer without concerns about pregnancy. Joe and Teresina were inspiring role models for me in this respect. They nurtured a very active sexual life into their eighties. Both were Buddhists who devoted their twilight years to creating "Temenos," a rustic haven for silent meditation retreats in western Massachusetts. Soon after retiring from the center they had created, Teresina was diagnosed with a prolapsed heart valve.

She and Joe visited several physicians, trying to evaluate the severity of her condition. The cardiologist outlined a long, depressing list of activities she would have to curtail.

"What about making love?" asked Teresina. "If I can't make love, I don't want to be here."

Despite the cardiologist's cautions, she and Joe made love in the mountain meadows surrounding their home. About three months after her diagnosis, Teresina was bedridden. Joe nursed her with the intense devotion of a grieving lover.

One afternoon Teresina muttered something to Joe. He bent forward, straining to hear every word.

"Oh, you old fool," laughed Teresina. "I was just bossing you around."

She continued to laugh, and died a few moments later, her lips still curved in a smile.

Reflections by Noreen Wessling

Born during Samhain in the beautiful city of Edinburgh, Scotland, Noreen immigrated to the United States at age fifteen. She attended the Art Academy of Cincinnati on scholarship and later earned a degree in psychology (magna cum laude) from the University of Cincinnati. Noreen created 7 Arts Studio, dedicated to inspiration, self-discovery, and contact with the inner spirit through creative activities. She has transformed her best dream journal sketches into Dream Treasure Cards, a deck of fifty cards to spark one's intuition. Noreen is also contributing editor and a popular author for Dream Network Journal.

I was in my early fifties when I went into menopause. I was exploring spiritual realms, primarily from a Gnostic perspective. In Gnosticism, learning from personal experience is most important, which is why dreaming has been so helpful to me.

I'd had years of tracking my inner promptings and knew that following that inner sense had more positive than negative outcomes in my life. When I began having symptoms and knew I was moving into perimenopause, I went to see my regular medical physician. He pushed me to start PremPro (Premarin and Provera combination).

"Let me think about it," I told him. He wanted me to start hormones immediately, but I didn't feel comfortable.

I paid attention to my dreams, incubated what I should do. My total knowing was *not* to follow the general trend. It didn't feel right to me. Period.

When I told my physician I wouldn't take the PremPro, he said, "Then I can't be your physician."

I had been seeing a chiropractor, Dr. Pittman, off and on for fifteen years. He focused on nutrition and testing. I went to see him, and he gave me Pro-Gest, a bio-identical progesterone cream. We also worked with nutrition and homeopathy, but Pro-Gest was the main focus. The Pro-Gest worked like a charm. I had some hot flashes, but they weren't horrible.

My mother said she never had any problems going through menopause. My aunt, who looked like me, had a horrible experience with menopause. She put on two hundred pounds. My aunt had always been thin. She was very depressed and took all of the drugs for menopause and depression. She died eighteen months after menopause. I looked at both relatives and decided to be like Mom.

I had always had terrible periods—irregular, heavy bleeding, severe cramping. I was also depressed around my periods. I didn't start menstruating until I was fifteen years old, which was very embarrassing, because all of my girlfriends had already started.

Menopause was the beginning of the best part of my life. There's no doubt about that. Life has been on an upward path since then. I was released from that great burden every month. I had an immense sense of freedom. Before, when I was having such bad menstrual periods, I would have to cancel things because I was so dragged out. I had a real sense of freedom without my periods.

It took about one or two years to stop bleeding. I ate "crone cookies," a recipe I got from Dr. Christiane Northrup, with herbs to support the menopausal transition. I continued to use the Pro-Gest.

I had several important turning points in my life. A couple of years before I started into perimenopause, I visited the Findhorn Foundation, a spiritual community in the north of Scotland. In 1990, I spent a week with Caroline Myss at Rio Caliente, a hot-springs retreat, in Mexico.

I began saving money so that I could return to Rio Caliente. In 1992, I went back. I had a whole month away from my normal lifestyle. So many things changed because I gave room in my life for things to appear.

A couple of weeks after I came back from Mexico, I began dream groups. The Pines Dream Sharers have been meeting monthly since then.

A month or two after returning from Mexico, I began dreaming about "getting down," getting dirty and primal. I became aware of drumming and wanted to try it. In 1992, I also began monthly drumming groups. I now offer an advanced class, "Learning Authentic African Rhythms," as well as the monthly drumming circle that has been ongoing since 1992.

A whole new level of creative energy was open to me after going through menopause. Before menopause, a lot of my creativity went into my periods. Lots of energy was directed to my children. Menopause, being at the Findhorn Foundation, and spending time with Caroline Myss changed where my creativity wanted to go. Before menopause, my creativity was more internal, more focused on family, children, and my personal art. After menopause, my creativity took an outward stroke, into the community.

A couple of years after menopause, I became very ill and almost died. I had severe pneumonia. I went back to my regular physician, who gave me antibiotics. I continued to worsen. Finally my husband, Dick, drove me to Dr. Pittman, the chiropractor. He saved me again, with herbs and homeopathic remedies.

I was having prolific dreams during the illness. Many of the dreams suggested I have a separate space, away from the house, for my own personal artwork. As soon as I began to feel better, Dick and I received an unexpected check, something to do with a stock we had, for $26,000. Dick spent exactly $26,000 building Seven Arts Studio.

It was like I was being rebuilt, regenerated after being so ill, and my husband was building the studio at the same time. 7 Arts Studio was supposed to be a personal art studio. We invited people for the opening of the studio on January 1, 1996.

Immediately the studio became a community building, not my personal art studio. Before, classes were held in the house. When the classes moved to the studio, they began expanding.

I had a dream ten years before the studio was built. A throng of people came to "The Pines" (the name my husband and I have given our home).

"We're seekers," said the people.

"This is private property," I told them.

"We're not leaving." They refused to budge.

"You have to."

"No. We're not going."

Finally I said, "OK, you can stay."

I dismissed the dream at the time. Later I realized 7 Arts Studio was a place for the community, not just my personal art.

Before menopause, I was much more an *inner* person, focused on family; personal art, and handwriting analysis, which I've been doing for thirty years. After menopause, I became a group person, a sharer in spite of myself. I became someone who was part of building something really good. I naturally felt drawn to share drumming, dreaming, and tai chi. Now other people are coming to teach too.

I've had a continuous expansion of my creative spirit since menopause. I've also had down times, like when I've come back from traveling in Europe and been sick. I return with lots of creative ideas though, too.

My advice for perimenopause: Find the deeper meaning in menopause for yourself. Research different cultures and discover how they viewed menopause. For my mom, in her contemporary culture, menopause was "the beginning of the end." For me, menopause was "the beginning of the beginning." Consider a more holistic approach for treating hot flashes. Medications may be good for some women, but they weren't for me. Menopause is part of life, part of who we are. Embrace it!

You may contact Noreen at: 7 Arts Studio, 5429 Overlook Road, Milford OH 45150; (513) 831-7045; Email: NoreenFW@cinci.rr.com; Website: www. creativespirit.net/noreens7artsstudio

Making Informed Choices about Hormone Replacement Therapy (HRT): Body Wisdom

Each woman has her own unique experience of menopause. Some women breeze through menopause while others struggle with a host of symptoms that range from unpleasant to disabling. Obviously the number and severity of symptoms influence a woman's decision about whether to take hormones, and for how long.

Making Choices that Suit Your Unique Health-care Needs

Both your personal and family medical history also have an important bearing on your health during perimenopause and menopause. Past alcohol intake, tobacco use, diet, and exercise heavily influence your current state of health. The lifestyle choices you make now can maintain, improve, or undermine your health. You have most control over the daily lifestyle decisions you make, decisions that are paramount in determining your overall well-being. Hormones can augment but never take the place of good lifestyle choices.

Are Your Symptoms Interfering with Your Life?

For women who have an exceptionally rough menopausal transition, hormone therapy can be a godsend. Only you can decide the severity of your symptoms and how adversely they are affecting your life. As you review the following list of possible menopausal symptoms from chapter 1, consider how these symptoms influence your life. Your family's, spouse's or coworkers' reactions to your condition are not as important as your own assessment. If a woman is concerned about lack of libido, for instance, I ask if the decrease in sexual desire is a problem for her or her mate. If she reports she used to enjoy sex and misses that connection with her mate, I am more concerned than if she tells me her mate doesn't really care about sex, but she thinks she "should."

Perimenopausal and Menopausal Symptom Questionnaire

For each symptom listed below, rate the severity of your symptoms, from 0 (nonexistent) to 5 (severe, that is, significantly interferes with your life).

- Hot flashes_____
- Night sweats_____
- Thinning hair_____
- Vaginal dryness _____
- Vaginal atrophy (thinning of vaginal tissue) _____
- Dry skin and hair _____
- Increased hair growth on face and body _____
- Memory lapses, especially short-term memory _____
- Insomnia _____
- Irritability, nervousness _____
- Anxiety _____
- Decreased sexual desire _____
- Depression _____
- Panic attacks _____
- Migraine headaches _____
- Osteoporosis _____
- Sore heels _____
- Urinary tract infections _____
- Sore breasts _____

SCORING YOUR QUESTIONNAIRE

How many "5s" (severe symptoms) did you score? If you have marked more than four symptoms as "severe," you may be a candidate for HRT.

You can return to this list every six to twelve months to reassess your journey through perimenopause into menopause. New symptoms may emerge while others change in severity or resolve. You will have a record of changes as you navigate this passage.

HRT for Symptomatic Relief

If you have low risk for osteoporosis (see assessment below) and want to take HRT for symptomatic relief only, you would most likely take hormones for six to eighteen months, not for the rest of your life. If you are taking HRT for symptoms alone and they have resolved, talk to your physician about how to slowly wean off the hormones.

Risks for Developing Osteoporosis

Osteoporosis is a bone disease marked by significant bone loss and increased risk of fracture. Over seventy-five million people in Europe, Japan and the United States suffer with osteoporosis, and the vast majority of this group are women.[1]

The World Health Organization defines osteoporosis as bone loss of more than 2.5 standard deviations (SD) below the average peak bone-mineral density for young adults. We will discuss testing bone mineral density (BMD) in more detail below.

The best way to safeguard against osteoporosis is to maximize bone health earlier in life. The higher your peak bone-mineral density between ages thirty-five and forty, the lower your risk of hip and other fractures later in life. Diet and exercise, which we will discuss more fully in chapters 10 and 11, are your best allies in preventing osteoporosis.

Fracture Risk and Bone Density

- Mild risk: bone density is 75–85% of young adults.

- Moderate risk: bone density is 65–75% of young adults.

- Moderate to severe risk: bone density is 55–65% of young adults.

- Severe risk: bone density is less than 55% of young adults.

Listed below are many factors that can influence bone density. The more risk factors you have, the more likely you are to develop osteoporosis.

- Personal health profile: female, fair skin, blue eyes, small body frame, slender. African American women, who tend to have higher peak bone-mineral density, are at lowest risk,[2] followed by Hispanic women. Asian and white women are at highest risk.[3]

- Late-onset menses[4]

- Missed menses. Women who miss up to half of their periods have 88 percent of the bone mass of normally menstruating women. Women who miss more than half their cycles have 69 percent of normal bone mass.[5]

- Family history of osteoporosis, particularly your mother

- Postmenopausal, because of changes in reproductive hormone levels

- Inadequate calcium intake, particularly in younger years

- Inactive lifestyle

- History of stress fractures

- An extended period of being confined to bed, in a wheelchair, or paralyzed

- Eating disorders, for example, anorexia nervosa[6]

- Certain medications, including anticonvulsants, isoniazid, furosemide, aluminum-containing antacids, cortisone and prednisone, tetracycline, heparin, prolonged high doses of thyroid

- Bowel diseases (for example, Irritable Bowel Syndrome, Crohn's), malabsorption syndrome, removal of part or all of the intestines, intestinal bypass for weight control

- Smoking tobacco, which lowers estrogen and vitamin C levels

- Moderate to high alcohol intake

- High dietary intake of caffeine, animal protein, sugar, sodium, phosphates (for example, carbonated soft drinks)

The three most important risk factors for developing osteoporosis are current use of an antiseizure medication, mother and maternal female relatives with a history of hip fracture, and inability to get up from a chair without using one's arms.[7]

IMPORTANT LAB TESTS FOR OSTEOPOROSIS

X-rays show bone deterioration only after you have lost 25 percent or more of the bone. Fortunately other tests more accurately detect bone-density changes at much earlier stages.

The dual energy X-ray absorptiometry (DEXA) is the best radiological test available to measure bone density of the lumbar (lower) spine and femoral neck (top of the thigh bone). The DEXA test uses a lower dose of radiation than an X-ray and takes less time than some of the other testing methods. The DEXA test is our current "gold standard" for measuring bone-mineral density.

Ultrasound of the heel is a great screening test for osteoporosis. Our skeletons are made of two types of bone: trabecular and cortical. The spine is made of 90 percent trabecular and 10 percent cortical bone, and the hip is half of each. The heel bone is 100 percent trabecular bone, which means the ultrasound test most accurately predicts the risk of heel and vertebral (spine) fracture. Because the ultrasound test cannot monitor cortical bone, any woman with abnormal ultrasound test results should be referred for a DEXA scan to more accurately assess her overall bone health.

WHEN SHOULD I HAVE A BONE-MINERAL DENSITY SCAN?

If you are at high risk for developing osteoporosis, consider having a baseline DEXA test between ages thirty-five and forty, when your bones should be at their peak density. If you already show significant loss at this early age, you could begin more aggressive treatment and possibly avert or reduce long-term bone loss.

If you have mild to moderate risk of osteoporosis, you may want to wait until your first year of menopause to have a bone-mineral-density scan. This baseline screening allows you to assess current bone health and track your progress over time. If you have high bone-mineral density, you may choose not to focus on lifestyle changes and supplements to maintain bone health. You can repeat the test in one to two years to see if you have maintained, increased, or lost bone-mineral density. Any bone loss would signal the need to pursue more aggressive treatment. If your first test shows significant bone loss, you may want to make lifestyle changes *and* take HRT. Repeat the DEXA scan every one to three years to assess the effectiveness of your treatment program. Ideally you would repeat the same type of bone-mineral-density test on the exact same machine; otherwise, you are comparing apples to oranges.

In chapter 9, we will discuss an additive program to support bone health.

What about HRT and Heart Disease?

Although many physicians have touted HRT as a way of lowering the risk of heart disease, very few recent studies have corroborated this claim. One of the major studies cited in favor of estrogen replacement therapy was a retrospective observational study, meaning researchers looked at past records (retrospective) and observed the relationship between HRT and heart disease. The study demonstrated that women who took HRT had lower risk of developing heart disease. The researchers failed to mention, however, that during the time period being reviewed, women were not given HRT if they had high blood pressure or any major risks for developing heart disease. The very fact they were given HRT indicated the women were at low risk for heart disease in the first place![8]

More recent research from the Heart and Estrogen/Progestin Replacement Study (HERS) suggests that estrogen- and progestin-replacement therapy actually increases the risk of having a stroke or heart attack by 50 percent during the first year of therapy. After that time, cardiovascular disease risk decreases.[9] After 4.1 years, the HERS study found that estrogen/progestin replacement had no effect in preventing coronary heart disease in postmenopausal women.

As mentioned in chapter 4, we do know that synthetic progestins cause spasms of coronary blood vessels, which may in turn increase risk of heart attack. For women who choose to take HRT, especially those concerned about heart disease, bio-identical progesterone is probably a better choice than synthetic progestins.

We certainly have much more to learn about hormones and cardiovascular disease. While waiting for further research information, my bias is to base HRT decisions on the severity of a woman's menopausal symptoms, her risk for developing osteoporosis, the results of a bone-mineral-density scan and any other necessary lab tests.

If you are considering taking HRT, refer back to chapter 4, p. XXX, for specific information about the "friendliest" types of hormone prescriptions.

Reevaluate Your Decision about HRT as Needed

Rather than offering a simple one-size-fits-all prescription for peri-menopausal and menopausal women ("Everyone should take HRT!" or "No one should take HRT!"), I encourage you to consider your past and current health history, the severity of your symptoms, and your family medical history when making this important decision. Revisit your conclusions about HRT as your health changes so that your choices match your current state of health.

DEVELOPING BODY WISDOM

How will I ever make appropriate decisions about what my body does or does not need, you may be wondering. Certainly hormone testing can provide information. Many physicians, though, review the tests and suggest dosing hormones to maintain reproductive-age levels of hormones after menopause. They see maintaining hormone levels as the "holy grail" of youth. As mentioned earlier, the number and severity of your symptoms are an important guide to evaluating your need for hormone replacement therapy. An equally important key is learning to listen to your own body wisdom.

My Body, My Earth

While on a ten-day silent Vipassana meditation retreat, our teacher mentioned how years of meditation had damaged his knee.

"I just kept going into the pain," he explained, "observing, watching, noticing how I liked or disliked the sensation. I was learning to observe the *sensation,* rather than call it 'pain.'"

Our teacher's story was a profound teaching about observing without labeling something as "good" or "bad." I appreciated the finely developed mindfulness, yet I was also distressed that he had used this skill to damage his body.

During the next sitting meditation period, I sank my attention deeply into my own body. I was amazed at the variety of sensations within my physical vehicle. I noticed how I retracted from neck and shoulder pain, and how I settled easily into areas that were relaxed and pliant. As I moved during walking meditation, I marveled at the coordination of muscles, tendons, nerves, and blood vessels to support my movements. I became more and more deeply aware of the miraculous physical creation I called "my body."

I was inspired during these meditations to more fully inhabit my body. "Here is my center of awareness," I thought. "All of these body sensations are profound anchors for my awareness. I can sink into the elements right here: water/blood, air; mineral/bone, fire/warmth, or coolness. I have my own planet right here, within me."

I realized that this miraculous "earth" body benefited from careful stewarding, just as the larger planet flourished with respectful attention. Overriding my body's distress signals, as Robert had with his knees, was just as damaging as overlooking the earth's devastation.

I walked into the dining room, wondering how I could communicate this understanding of my own body as a microcosm of the earth to our teacher.

"Robert," I said, approaching him as he was scraping his lunch dishes. He turned to face me.

"I want to share something with you." I placed my hand over his heart and looked into his eyes. "This is your earth."

I know in retrospect that my words had much more power than my usual utterances, as I had been in silence for several days. The longer I refrain from speaking, the more power my words transmit.

"What?" he asked. "You mean like the earth, loving your Mother . . ."

I looked intently into his eyes. I kept my hand on his chest. "Robert, this is your earth."

A look of recognition shot through his eyes. "Oh, my body, the earth . . ." He burst into tears. We stood for a few moments, hugging and crying.

I offer you the same "transmission" of understanding. Place your hand on your heart. (I would place my hand on your heart if I was there.) This is your earth. Please say it out loud. "This is my earth."

Deeply understanding that your body *is* your earth can profoundly alter your relationship with your body as well as with the larger spheres of life around you. This body is the stuff of the earth. This body is the part of the earth for which you are most directly responsible. Taking care of this body automatically links you with taking care of the planet Earth. The foods that best nourish this body-earth, for example (local, organic, whole foods), also nourish the planet Earth. Foods that undermine body health, such as highly processed, sugary foods trucked or flown over long distances, also destroy the planet Earth. Movements that best support this body-earth (walking, dancing,) also support the planet Earth. Lack of movement—for example, driving cars and flying in planes—undermines our stamina and pollutes the planet Earth.

This body is my earth, my personal "planet" that will carry me through the orbit of my life.

Honoring this body-earth begins to develop what I call "body wisdom." Deep attention to the cycles within our own bodies begins to link us with the larger cycles of creation. The very cycles whispering in this body also inform the movement of planets, asteroids, and stars. The same whirling of life informs subatomic particles. From the least to the greatest, from the most expansive to the most elemental, the stuff of creation links us with the mysteries of life. This body is the Word made flesh. Spirit breathes your inspiration, and spirit drums the rhythm of your heart. This body is Creator's hand within your own.

Diamond Body

Qigong (pronounced "tsee gong") is the practice of cultivating qi, or life force and vitality, in our bodies. Some spiritual traditions promise a better life in the hereafter. The physical world is illusory, a distraction from the "true" sphere of disembodied spirituality. Practitioners devote their spirituality to negating their physical forms and instead focusing on the unseen realms of spirit.

In contrast, qigong practitioners devote themselves to bringing more and more spirit into the world of physical form, right here, right now. Instead of escaping physicality to embrace spirit, they bring body and spirit together, uniting heaven and earth through their movements and awareness.

"Enlightenment" is literally increased light in our physical bodies. Enlightenment comes *through* our bodies, not despite them. This light, described in almost every spiritual tradition, is a byproduct of profound awakening. I used to giggle when I saw medieval paintings of the saints with golden halos around their heads. The images looked so contrived, so "kitchy." Now I understand that the artists were attempting to depict the golden, or sometimes peach-colored, light that surrounds those of us who are deeply awake, who serve as conduits for bringing more light into the world.

Professor Hui Xian Chen, my qigong teacher, told the story of a young man about five hundred years ago, who at the age of twenty-four went into the mountains to live in seclusion. He devoted his life to practicing qigong and meditation. He passed quietly at the age of 126. No one knew that he had died.

Three years later a general passed by and discovered the body of this deceased monk. The body was still in perfect condition. In many Asian traditions, when a practitioner reaches such an enlightened state that the body remains unblemished after death, he or she is said to have achieved the "diamond body."

To honor the monk, the general built a special seat for the monk's body to sit on, and a simple building to house the relic. Many people came to visit the site. Eventually other monks came to meditate and live at the site. The body still contained tremendous energy. Just being in the proximity of this "diamond body" awakened people. Sitting near the body healed many ailments.

The body remained at the site for over five hundred years, still in perfect condition. In 1966, during the Cultural Revolution in China, the local monks were afraid that the Red Guard would destroy the diamond body. Mao was determined to rid China of "superstition," which included all spiritual practices and beliefs. The Red Guard destroyed many temples and holy sites during this time.

The local monks buried the body deep in the earth next to the temple. Thankfully, the Red Guard overlooked this simple monastery deep in the mountains.

Ten years later, at the end of the Cultural Revolution, the monks dug up the relic. Even after burial, the diamond body was still in good condition.

Christ's Body Is My Body

The Catholic Church also recognizes this physical state of enlightenment that preserves the body after death, and refers to them as "The Incorruptibles." After death, the bodies do not decompose. The Incorruptibles continue to perform miracles, blessing pilgrims and local worshippers long after their "death." Several of the Catholic saints were Incorruptibles; others were not. Being an Incorruptible is not a condition of sainthood. St. Francis' body, for example, decomposed, while his spiritual companion Clare was an Incorruptible.

Symeon the New Theologian (949–1022) beautifully describes his experience of union with divinity through his physical body:

We awaken in Christ's body
as Christ awakens our bodies,
and my poor hand is Christ, He enters
my foot, and is infinitely me.

I move my hand, and wonderfully
my hand becomes Christ, becomes all of Him
(for God is indivisibly
whole, seamless in His Godhood).

I move my foot, and at once
He appears like a flash of lightning.
Do my words seem blasphemous?—Then
open your heart to Him

and let yourself receive the one
who is opening to you so deeply.
For if we genuinely love Him,
we wake up inside Christ's body

where all our body, all over,
every most hidden part of it,
is realized in joy as Him,
and He makes us, utterly, real,

and everything that is hurt, everything
that seemed to us dark, harsh, shameful,
maimed, ugly, irreparably
damaged, is in Him transformed

and recognized as whole, as lovely,
and radiant in His light
we awaken as the Beloved
in every last part of our body.[10]

Creating from the Womb

As women, we obviously create babies from our wombs. Gradually I've come to realize that the womb is the most potent source of any creation, whether physical or nonphysical.

During a recent silent retreat, I was on my moon-time and bleeding heavily. I had never before had the opportunity to sit and walk in stillness, deeply observing the internal shifts that come with menstrual bleeding. I was often drawn, almost irresistibly, to focus on my womb. Pain was not the magnet, but rather a powerful creative force.

I began to see that any act of creation directed from the womb will always be life-giving. The outcome may also be a surprise. I can't control everything that comes from the womb. I don't always expect the "children" who come; they may be very different from what I have envisioned.

The veil between the worlds is thinnest at the onset of menses. If I am still, perhaps I will glimpse the Divine. If I am immersed in work and the endless details of daily living, I will likely miss spirit's whisperings.

According to some archeologists, the earliest blood offerings in the temples were likely women's menstrual blood, not animal sacrifices. These cultures understood the power of women, who could bleed and not die. When young women held this blood inside, they created babies from that blood. When elderly women carried their blood, they grew wisdom within their wombs.

Christ understood the blood mysteries, the miracle of blood and body, the very foundation of creation, when he offered bread and wine at the Last Supper: "'Take this [bread]; this is my body.' Then he took a cup, and having offered thanks to God he gave it to them; and all drank from it. And he said, 'This is my blood, the blood of the covenant, shed for many.'"[11] He was creating a way for us to ingest his spirit into our bodies—the Word, and the *mystery*, becoming one with our flesh.

Listening Deeply to the Body

How can we fine-tune this ability to listen deeply to body wisdom? Almost always the body whispers before it shouts. Body language can be subtle. If I am alert to quiet communications, the body may not need more desperate signals. Dreams, meditations, and energy awareness can hone our ability to listen to body signals.

Of course we also have the choice to override body signals. When a cold develops, for example, our bodies often want rest. The body craves quiet, inward time.

"Oh, I'm too busy for that," we often tell ourselves. "I've got to get to work, take care of the kids, facilitate this important meeting. I can't just go to bed."

We can take antibiotics or other medications and "power through" the illness. In the short term, we save time. In the long run, though, our bodies are often more vulnerable to future illnesses.

A family friend described going to see his physician for a bad cold. In his mid-eighties, this seasoned family physician was nearing retirement. The physician handed my friend a prescription for antibiotics.

"I really don't care whether or not you fill this," he told my friend. "What's most important is that you go to bed and stay in bed for twenty-four hours after the fever breaks. If you get up too soon, you will be back here in six weeks for another prescription of antibiotics."

This sage elder knew that overriding the body's need for rest would weaken the immune system and make the body more vulnerable to future infections.

Listening to the body and heeding its signals can augment vitality. Herbs and homeopathic medicines catalyze the body's ability to heal itself, rather than suppressing or overriding symptoms. Working appropriately with homeopathic medicines and herbs can improve our constitutions, leaving us stronger at the end of the illness.

Dreams as a Source of Healing

Dreams may offer wisdom about the cause and/or the cure for an illness. Noreen Wessling's interview is a powerful testament to the healing power of dreams (see pp. XXX). Phyllis Rodin dreamed about a cure for a poisonous spider bite. She was in the hospital in India, and her physicians had given up hope that she would survive the night. "That night," Phyllis remembers, "I dreamt I was reading a book. On page 64, the book said that American Indians drank their urine to cure themselves of poisonous bites. I woke in the night, urinated in a glass, and drank the urine. In the morning, the doctors were shocked to find me alive. I continued to drink my urine and walked out of the hospital a few days later."

Thankfully Phyllis trusted this nocturnal guidance, despite the fact it was far outside her own cultural experience. An interesting aside: although

Phyllis's dream cited Native American traditions, India also has a long history of medically supervised urine therapy.

Sometimes the dream itself is a powerful healing. One patient, a rough-and-tumble jokester who worked as a local janitor, came to me for treatment of chronic heel pain. While on the table, he shared a profound experience he had had some thirty years before. His doctor at the time had diagnosed him with diabetes. That night he left his body shortly after falling asleep and spent the night talking with Jesus. Christ shared many profound insights with him during the night. When he woke in the morning, the janitor was cured of diabetes. The symptoms have never returned.

Healing Meditations

Insights about healing may come during meditations. Years ago I spent a winter week fasting and meditating on Iona, a sacred island off the west coast of Scotland. During that time, I "heard" in meditation that I was to rub moistened salt into the soles of my feet. I thought the information strange, but dutifully rubbed salt into my feet during my showers that week. Years later, while studying naturopathic medicine, I discovered the "salt glow" treatment, a time-honored therapy that supports detoxification of the body.

Below is a meditation to explore listening to different aspects of your body. Approach this meditation as you might a date with a new friend: you are getting to know each other, body and mind, in a new way.

MEDITATION

Sit in a comfortable location, with your spine straight. Remove as many distractions as possible (for example, phone off the hook, kids in bed, and so on). Take several deep breaths, allowing your breath to move all the way into your lower abdomen.

Place your attention at the very base of the trunk of your body, approximately between your vaginal and rectal openings. Some women perceive this energetic center between their ovaries. The specific location is not as important as listening to this region of your body. What does this area feel like? Do you sense warmth, coolness, lightness, and/or pressure? Do any images come to your mind? What does this area have to say to you? What wisdom does it have to offer? What does this region need? Take your time. The body speaks at its own pace, in its own way. You may "see" pictures in your mind's eye, feel different sensations, or sense words. Write down anything that you want to remember in your journal.

Move your attention now to an area about two finger-breadths below your navel, right in the center of the body. In qigong, this area is called "lower dan tien," or "lower burner." This is the very center of the body. If you placed a pin directly through this point from front to back, the body would rotate evenly around that pin. Again, note sensations in this area. Ask for wisdom. Inquire if this area needs anything to achieve optimal health. Listen deeply to the body's response. Write down your observations.

Shift your attention upward to the solar plexus area. Note the sensations in this area. Do you feel radiant here, or contracted? What do you see, sense, and feel in this region? What wisdom does the solar plexus have to offer? What does this area need for full health and vitality? Note anything you want to remember in your journal.

Move to the heart region, in the center of the chest. What do you feel here? What images, memories, or sensations greet you? What wisdom does the heart have to offer? What does this area need to flourish? Make notes in your journal.

Place your attention in the throat region. What sensations do you have in the throat? Is this area free and relaxed, or constricted? What images, words, or feelings arise as you focus on this area? What wisdom does the throat have to offer? What does the throat need for optimal health? Again, record your observations.

Focus now on the center of the forehead. What does this area feel like? What do you sense as you listen to this area? What wisdom does this part of your body have to offer? What would allow this area to flourish? Make notes in your journal.

Shift your awareness to the top of the head. What sensations do you note here? Do any memories or words arise? What wisdom does the top of the head have to offer? What does this area need for optimal health? Write your observations in your journal.

Move your awareness to the soles of your feet, just behind the ball of the foot. How does this area feel? What do you sense, hear, or see in this part of your body. This is your most immediate connection with the earth. What wisdom does this region have to offer? What do your feet need for optimal health? Note anything you want to remember in your journal.

Finally, scan your body from head to toe. Does your body feel any different than when you started this meditation? Are any areas calling for further attention?

Follow the movement of breath in and out of your body for a few minutes. Let your body settle into this relaxed awareness.

When you are ready, open your eyes and record any final observations.

You can return to this meditation over and over again. Like "dates" with a friend or new lover, you will discover new aspects of the body each time you practice deep listening. Regular contact and intent listening will deepen this blossoming relationship with your physical temple.

Riding the Rapids

Carol Bridges notes that menopause is one of two times in our lives when we receive "spiritual boosts" so that we can create what we want in the next phase of our lives. We are riding a much stronger, fuller energetic current, like easing from a lazy creek into a turbulent river. The menopausal signals in our body can be strong, and may require moment-by-moment calibration. Kathleen Luiten describes the need to learn how to tune "up" or "down" the energy in the body, much like moving up and down the keyboard of a piano, to meet the body's shifting needs. When the current runs faster, we run faster. When the current slows, we slow. The (sometimes damnable) challenge of menopause is that the currents can shift within minutes.

Several cultures have developed what I call "body wisdom technologies" to help develop body awareness and flexibility to meet these shifting currents. Both yoga and qigong are ancient technologies designed to support physical, mental, emotional, and spiritual health. More advanced qigong practices incorporate spontaneous movements. At this stage, the qi itself becomes a guide for restoring normal function in the body.

Ideally you would find a teacher to guide your learning. Often a teacher can illuminate blind spots and facilitate our progress. While studying qigong, I would return to teacher trainings after months of practice, certain I had perfected the form. My teacher would make tiny adjustments and radically increase the energy flow in the body. Gradually I learned to welcome rather than resent these corrections, as they increased the qi in my body.

Trying to learn qigong without a qualified instructor can lead to "deviation," or abnormal qi flow in the body. Incorrectly practicing qigong can actually cause rather than cure illness. There are thousands of qigong forms, both ancient and contemporary, and only a few are safe to learn on your own. Rather than learning from a video, DVD, or book, find a teacher who can guide you in practicing qigong safely and effectively.

Learning directly from a teacher, no matter what art or form you study, links you with a lineage of instructors. You receive a living transmission of the teachings. When I practice qigong, I am aware of a long lineage of teachers and students who have preceded me. I stand with over eight thousand years of dedicated practitioners behind me.

You may have had the same experience saying a mantra, the Lord's Prayer, or the rosary: you say these prayers with the strength of nuns, monks, and parishioners, all of those who have ever uttered those prayers over millenia. If you are praying within a living tradition, your voice joins a river of millions of others who are saying, or who have ever uttered, those prayers.

Books can expand your mind, but only direct experience can immerse you in the river of living tradition.

With so many choices available for developing body wisdom, which one should you choose? Trust your own body to give you feedback. You may have a profound sense of peace as you learn, or have a deep experience while practicing. Perhaps your heart will pound with excitement.

You may also begin to notice changes in your body. Is your health improving? Do you have more energy, more patience, more peace in your life? Does this practice open your heart as well as strengthen your body?

Listen deeply to your body for cues about what systems or forms are best for you. Be aware that your body may need different kinds of support during certain periods of your life. The form that was appropriate when you were twenty-five years old may not be the most beneficial when you are fifty-five. Again, listen for the body's wisdom about what is best for you now.

Earth/Body Wisdom

Beyond preventative listening, body wisdom can also crack open a whole new way of perceiving and participating in life. As mentioned earlier, observing the body can deepen awareness in meditation. Profound observation of the particulars in our body can also turn us "inside out," catapulting awareness into much broader spheres.

Professor Chen describes how years of qigong practice has attuned her with much larger planetary cycles. That awareness is a double-edged sword, because developing profound earth/body sensitivity also means being attuned to the earth's imbalances. In the short term, these perceptions can be unsettling. In the long run, however, this body awareness can save lives.

While living in Australia, a friend who had spent years living with Australian aboriginal people told me a story that helped me understand the depth of most traditional indigenous people's connection with the land. He described how a few years before the aboriginal people of the Central Territory had quietly left a certain region. Even ants vacated the area. The white Europeans continued their mining excavations, oblivious to the exodus of almost every living creature. Two weeks later a tremendous earthquake rocked the area. The miners lost a huge land-moving machine that toppled into a deep crack opened by the earthquake.

Linking with the cycles in this physical body automatically bonds you with much larger circles of life. The moon pulls the water in our cells as strongly as the tides of the ocean. The planets keep their orbits as faithfully as the trajectories of subatomic particles. We are dancing to the same drum, vibrating to the same harmonies as the larger cycles of creation. Listening attentively to our physical vehicle can deepen rather than detract from our spiritual lives.

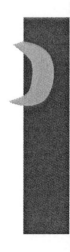

Reflections by Kathleen Luiten

Kathleen Luiten is an American mystic connecting with earnest students worldwide through teleconferences, workshops, and silent retreats. Her teachings blend depth practices from Eastern and Western lineages including Tibetan Tantric Buddhism, depth psychology, and the mystery schools. She shares practices and transmission for awakening "enlightenment in form"—living human life fully informed by the seed vibration Om, the divine energy permeating all form and formlessness.

Entering perimenopause and menopause has been a relatively easy transition for me, moving through yet another stage of change as I progress through the decades of my life. The transition was easier for me because I had already experienced significant physical and spiritual challenges and learned to let my body guide me through such times. Beginning in my late teens, I had a series of infections that brought me very close to death. Years of illness and a difficult journey back to wellness taught me much about living in a body as it changes its patterns and needs. What I learned from my body transformed my entire life. Initially I was a very resistant student of her wisdom, but eventually I deepened my understanding of what I now call "body wisdom." Following that wisdom has led me to the most fulfilling experiences of my life. Each of us, transitioning through a major stage of our lives, has a similar opportunity to resist the change or to develop a new self in harmony with what has come. I will share just a few of my stories from those years when I first learned to let go of my resistance and discovered the harmony that my body created for me.

To provide some context, you should know that when I was young I planned to be a physicist. I loved the world of the mind, mathematics, and especially theoretical physics. I showed some promise as a budding scientist in college and intended a career that would lead to academia and years of living inside the beautiful formulas that might one day evolve to describe the wholeness of our relational universe. That was my plan as I started my first year at the university, but my mind's intention and my spirit's passion were derailed as my body—intervening rather harshly—set me on a dramatically different course.

As soon as I began college I had a series of infections that continued for over four years. I saw many, many doctors as I was shuffled through the medical system, awaiting a scientific "cure." Finally one specialist, yet another doctor in the long chain of experts I had seen, reviewed my chart and said, "Hmm, I see that you've been chronically ill for over three years."

"I have?" I said, surprised by this news. This was a small but genuine beginning of my awakening to body wisdom. I realized that I was not paying attention to my own life and was waiting for a doctor to fix my problem. I realized that I wasn't taking responsibility for my physical condition.

This specialist went on to do more examinations and gave me the first of the many diagnoses I received. Apparently my physical condition was something that didn't fit the textbook cases. I saw a string of specialists over the next year and a half, each giving me a different tentative diagnosis and recommending more tests. So the scientist in me eventually accepted the fact that the medical experts really couldn't determine what was causing my illness. The only consensus was that there was a problem with my immune system, and that they did not have any effective treatment for it.

After my mini-awakening, realizing I needed to be responsible for my own health, I began to research. I improved my nutrition, took supplements, and tried to exercise my very weak body.

What I was doing didn't make much difference, and the constant infections continued. In my early twenties I became critically ill. Doctors could offer palliative care, but I was told that there was nothing that would cure me. I was "terminal." Again I saw a round of specialists, each curious about my case. At that point I was bedridden and very limited in what I could do. I had refused to take any more drugs and all of my vital statistics were below normal, life-sustaining levels. My blood pressure on a good day was 50/30. Respiration was typically about 3 breaths per minute. If I sat up, I passed out. Apparently I had no measurable adrenal function. Physicians would examine me with curiosity because they couldn't really explain why I was still alive. The last time I was in the hospital, they said it would be a matter of days at the most, and it was just a deathwatch.

Obviously I am alive to share this story, so I did not die in that hospital bed. Too weak to stand up, I asked my boyfriend to take me out of there. I just didn't want to be in the hospital anymore. If they couldn't do anything for me, I wanted to be at home. This was another small attempt to maintain personal responsibility for my life even if there wasn't much left of it.

My boyfriend agreed. He had to carry me out of the hospital because the nurses refused to bring in a wheelchair. I was insistent that I leave immediately, so I signed papers while I was in his arms, saying I relieved them of all responsibility. He carried me to the car and drove me back home to die.

About three days after I returned home, according to my boyfriend, I drew my last breath. He was premed, not a doctor, but he had some knowledge of the body's process. He checked for a pulse in several locations and used a mirror in front of my mouth to see if there was any breath. He observed no pulse or visible breath for over twenty minutes. Then he called the coroner.

Meanwhile, I was having a very different experience. I remember being out of body, and calmly looking down at it lying in the bed. I was not going into the light. It wasn't anything like that. It felt *normal* to be where I was. I knew I could easily move beyond the realm of earth and that felt normal, too. With some years of hindsight I now know that I had always been conscious in that level of my Self—that's where I'd really been living while I was sleepwalking through much of my earthly existence.

So as I was calmly looking down at my body from a great distance, I had this sense of being where I had always been, and this wasn't special or different in any way at all from being in my body. I was exactly the same, but couldn't walk or smell or do any of the things we do through our body.

Then I had a very strong sense of how stupid I had been. I remember thinking, "I've used this body just like I've used my car." I'd had my first car when I went to college. I'd driven it, and driven it, figuring I could get new parts or even get a new car when I need it. But the doctors couldn't repair my body the way the mechanic fixed my car.

I had my first great awakening in that moment when out of my body: "Oh, the body is a living thing, and *living* things can't be used like that. They don't function the same way." It took dying to make me realize what living really is.

As I looked at my dead body, I had the sense of having wasted this life. I was very comfortable where I was, didn't have any sense of unfinished business to make me return. But where I was is what I always experienced. The body, living in the body, was the special opportunity. I decided that if I could, I was going to try to come back into it. *If* I could. And then I would really try to live the life of this body, because I finally realized that I had really blown a unique opportunity.

So I literally willed myself back into my body. I actually remember it vividly, forcing a breath into my body for the first time. The act of will was something from my spirit, not my mind. And the effort was so much that I can't put it into words. The closest I can come to describing that first breath is to imagine you have a house sitting on your chest and you have to lift that house with your lungs to inhale. It was impossible. Yet I put all of my consciousness into coming back into the body, and it created that first breath.

When I inhaled, my boyfriend reports it was like a death rattle. He was shocked. Then there wasn't any breath for quite awhile. And then there was another breath. I remember trying to work the lungs like bellows, with all of my consciousness focused on them. I was willing to be alive again. After three or four more breaths I was able to open my eyes, and I was back.

If I lifted my head, I passed out. I was still just barely alive. After awhile

I was stable enough that my boyfriend could help me sit up. As soon as I could manage to speak, I said to him, "You need to take me to the doctor."

All of what had happened, and what was about to happen, led me to recognize that my body did not match the scientific model. This body didn't function on a logical, fact-based system. I was alive, just as I had been sick, without reasonable explanation. So I, the would-be scientist, had to surrender to the evidence: science was not the path to healing my body.

What soon followed my return to physical form was equally amazing and life defining. Within a week or so, I was able to stand up and walk. I went to a doctor and got some advice, and something that registered as a bit of wisdom, too. First he said, "You're dying, and I can't do anything about it," which was the same thing that all the doctors had said. And then he said, "The only way I know that will help you get better is to exercise." I laughed, because I could barely even stand up. The doctor knew I couldn't walk out of his office, let alone walk miles and climb hills as he was suggesting. He said, "I know it seems impossible. But it is your only chance." And something in that message registered as wisdom in me. My body, using my body to bring back my health, was my only chance. Now if I could just manage to do it!

About ten days later, I got a ride to a friend's house so that I could visit her before she died. While I was in the hospital I had been told that my friend had some kind of inoperable cancer. I didn't know anything else about her situation except that her physicians were doing everything possible to give her a few more months of life, and she was continuing to "battle the cancer." When I arrived, someone who was helping to care for her asked me if I would join in doing a little soothing massage. I had never given a massage—and was still very weak myself—so I just stood next to her, extending my hands and waiting for a sense of what kind of touch would be good for my friend.

And then the walls of science came tumbling down forever for me. I still can't say I believe what happened, but three of us all witnessed the impossible: little translucent white gobs emerged from my friend's body on strands attached to my fingers! I never touched her. I just felt drawn to move my hands over her belly and felt heat even with my hands more than a foot away. It felt too hot as I moved closer to her body, so I stopped and was waiting for her caretaker to show me how to do the massage. Then I looked at my hands, saw these balls, and shook them off. The balls bounced along the floor and disappeared. I thought I had hallucinated—maybe my out-of-body experience had provided too little oxygen to my brain—until I saw the faces of the other two women, both wide-eyed and staring at the spot where those gobs of whatever had vanished. Whoa! This was even stranger than being out-of-body and coming back to life. What was this?

My own illness had absorbed my attention for many months, so I had no idea what kind of cancer was consuming her body. I didn't know that my friend had multiple tumors in her abdomen. And what happened, according to the doctors who examined her the next day, was a spontaneous healing. All of her tumors were gone. She had been examined the day before her "massage," and then again the day after. She and her caretaker described what had happened, and her doctors wanted to meet me.

My world had turned inside out. I had no frame of reference for anything like spiritual healing and had no idea how it had happened. I remember hearing them bubble over with excitement, saying "You removed the tumors! They're gone!" All I could think was that I better not shake hands with anyone because I might remove a bone. And I was still barely alive, in need of a spontaneous healing myself. The last thing I wanted was any public exposure or distraction from my commitment to try to live in this body. So I went home, had friends put my clothes in my car, drove away, and never saw or talked to any of them again.

That move was the real beginning of my journey into body wisdom. I realized that in just a few short weeks I had experienced two truly phenomenal events. First I had apparently willed myself back to life after "dying," and then I had apparently witnessed and may have caused the tumors that were killing my friend to disappear from her body. Each one was undeniable. And each one was completely outside my current realm of understanding. I, in my little scientific mind, was being *forced* to acknowledge that the something outside of the scientific and medical model, outside of logic, and outside of everything I had been taught to consider as part of reality, could impact the body on a physical level. So my current understanding was obviously wrong. Reality was not what I believed it to be.

Academia hadn't given me the right answer, so I designed my own course of study. I didn't look to books, and I didn't look to other teachers. What had initiated my awakening had occurred in *me* and in my life. I didn't know what meditation was, but I started meditating. I had been meditating all my life, and I didn't realize it. Years later I found out what I was doing was called "meditation."

What I started doing was going deep within myself and trying to "figure it out." That's what I thought I was doing, using my mind, yet I knew that I couldn't really think about it. I had to sense the truth in a different way. And information came pouring into my conscious whenever I opened to it.

I began literally seeing my DNA. I watched what goes on in cells, and all sorts of things. I was still very skeptical, but having just lived through two reality-bending experiences, I realized I seemed to have a gift or an ability that had nothing to do with the ordinary education to which I'd been exposed.

I continued to explore this inner realm of information because I had come back into this body to *live* and was still considered terminally ill. I was trying to solve what was going on in my body that doctors hadn't been able to help me with. Many years passed before I finally understand what had made me sick. I had to open to new models for understanding bodies and life itself.

The Eastern model of the human energy system, including the aura and chakras that are now familiar terms throughout the world, was a useful tool for understanding and describing the work that I needed to do for my own healing. I discovered that the primary cause of my illness was sensory overload. I was born "wide open," a full-blown empath, that is I felt all the things that were around me—people, animals, even rivers and mountains. I had known this ability to feel from the time I was a child. I had thought everybody was like that. Now I know it is very rare and usually such children die young or become very ill as adults. Well, I did fit the second pattern!

When I moved to the dormitory at college, I was overloaded with sensory input all day and all night. My body showed the signs of the stress, and even after I moved it couldn't recuperate. My energy system was overloaded. Life was just too intense for me. My nervous system was over-stimulated, and that overload had thrown my body off. I needed to find a way to be less impacted by what was coming into me.

Sure enough, as I started to shift my sensitivity, I got healthier and healthier. I felt that what had seemed impossible was indeed possible. I really had to listen within myself, to both my body and my spirit. I had to listen to the *wisdom*—not just the obvious signals of change or discomfort in my body, but something deeper and more subtle. That inner sense or wisdom helped me to interpret my body's signals and understand the context unique to me, in this moment of life. As I grew stronger and trusted my own health, I began to work with others seeking to grow in their understanding of life's mystery.

This same access to body wisdom has guided me in working with others with their body wisdom. Each body has its own voice. We can learn so much from other people's experiences, the experiences that are shared here in this book and what other friends will share of their experiences. But my most important message to those experiencing any transition is listen to your *own* body and spirit. And don't allow body and spirit to become separate like I did! Look back at your own journey through previous transitions: a relationship ending, a job changing, puberty or illness. Your awakening and insight will come from your own journey. Just reflect on a past illness that your body recovered from and assume that your body was speaking about its own balance, trying to guide you to that recovery.

I needed the difference between wisdom and information shoved down my throat, because I was boxed into the logical model of a scientist. But my body defied science. I couldn't deny it. I had evidence. My experience broke the box. Then all I had to do was look inside, and discover that I am a wonderful vessel of intuition.

When I first had physical energy, when I drove away and never saw anybody of that group again, I went off where no one knew me. After about three months, I went out into nature and fasted for the first time in my life. I was at the stage in the fast when it became a water fast and decided I wanted to sit at the foot of a giant sequoia tree for the nine days of my water fast. I had the juice of two oranges in those nine days; otherwise it was pure water.

I gained forty-eight pounds in those nine days. I wouldn't have believed it, would have suspected a fast-induced hallucination, had a friend not been witness to it. So again my body was defying ordinary reality. At least now that felt more familiar to me!

I had been quite thin because I had been very ill. Now I was *fat*. I looked like the Pillsbury Doughboy. When I started the fast, I had been able to walk slowly. I had built up to walking half a block. And then I had to sit down and rest at least ten or twenty minutes. When I came home from the nine day fast, I went walking around the town I lived in, and I walked over five miles. It was just shocking to me. How could my muscles do that, after having atrophied for almost four years?

I looked at my reflection in a big window as I walked by, and I didn't even recognize myself because I was fifty pounds bigger. I had been about 110 pounds, and now I was about 160 pounds. I was almost half again that size, a big bulking hulk. I glanced at that figure, and my immediate response was, "That is *alive*." So I broke through that whole attitude many women have that being fat isn't good. It was just, "Wow! I'm alive. I'm *alive*."

Only years later did I truly understood the impact of my body's intervention. Instead of following the familiar, measurable path of scientific study that I had planned, I was catapulted into the unfamiliar and immeasurable realm of intuition and spirit. Not an easy journey for someone who thrives on formulas and logic! My experiences have led me to a life of work rooted in the immeasurable and invisible mystery of our existence, taking me from physics into the very meta physics of our universe. The lessons of my body have been my greatest teacher in this awakening.

Approaching menopause has been a relatively easy passage for me spiritually and physically because I had already experienced much more dramatic physical challenges. These challenges opened me to learning through my body, without holding any dominating belief that could distort my body's experience. I developed body wisdom. My experience was not one I would ever choose consciously—too much suffering!—but it has given me life beyond anything I had imagined possible.

I came from the scientific model with no belief in God or Soul. Through my serious illness and much physical pain I learned that we are truly spirit, spirit *informing* our body! And I learned that our body informs spirit as well. Spirit is learning and growing through its communion with this physical body. Ha! Body teaching spirit—that concept was quite different from most of the religious teachings surrounding me, which depicted body and nature as things to be controlled or overcome. Instead I found that there is no hierarchy between body and spirit, between nature and divinity. Eastern mysticism has long described the inseparable nature of the Yang and Yin; Sufi mystics speak of the All and the Nothingness as one and the same. I experienced this right here, in this simple female body by listening to her voice as my spirit and body journeyed together.

My physical life is still definitely a work in progress. I continue to find some things difficult to balance and I have much yet to learn. My life has taught me to open to the unknowable and allow the impossible.

And it has allowed me to learn a great deal about how to access our own body wisdom.

When I knew that my reflections on life's transitions would be included in this book I asked myself, "What is the best gift can I offer here? What do I know that seems to help virtually everyone in transition?"

The two best tools I've found that help most people to access body wisdom, and any form of wisdom, are deep meditation and smooth, repetitive exercise. Your meditation can be in the form of prayer, journaling, or a more traditional meditation practice, as long as you are consistent and take your focus into the depths of that experience. The physical exercise needs to be aerobic and repetitive, something like brisk walking or running, swimming laps or using an elliptical machine.

Meditation without movement can allow us a greater depth in our opening. Meditation or single mindedness while moving vigorously allows an integration with our body that can inform our spirit in different ways. It is really a lovely process to experience, breathing deeply and nurturing both body and spirit with mindfulness. I encourage you to settle into a routine of quiet, deep meditation and regular, mindful aerobic exercise. Use it as a moving meditation, opening to your intuition and getting into your zone of body wisdom.

After the experiences I had in my early twenties, menopause was not a major event for me. I had already faced death; I had developed body wisdom. Menopause, puberty, aging, or any kind of body transition can be a time of particularly deep insight and growth for each of us. The body's voice may be easier to hear during these transitions. We can each find new kinds of vitality and meaning if we are able to listen to the voice of our body's process and sustain our relationship of body and spirit as we change through life.

This small female body has been my most significant teacher as I have worked to drop the veils of ego and attachments, to live fully awakened in spirit within this body's form. I am grateful indeed for the teachings of my body, the *body wisdom* I have absorbed and now share through my work and my life.

My stories may seem dramatic, more the stuff of movies that usual life. Your stories are no less significant even if their voices are softer. It took strong, hot spices to awaken me. If yours are more subtle or sweet, so much the better to learn and enjoy!

For further information, please visit Kathleen's website: www.KathleenLuiten.com.

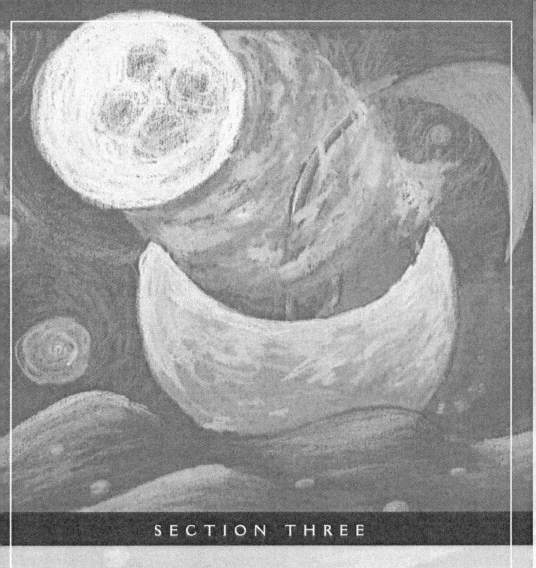

FOLLOWING the RIVER

Prelude to Section Three

The river winds through the mountains, dropping as the rocky shelves give way along the mountain's flanks. We haul the boat onto a small, sandy beach. River Woman motions me to follow her.

A path follows the river, then stops abruptly in a circle of rocks. I approach the barrier cautiously. Suddenly my stomach drops, like a driver cresting and dropping over an unexpected hill in the darkness.

In front of me the land drops away, and I see only open sky and an enormous stretch of water far below. The "river" we have been paddling free-falls almost a thousand feet below where I stand. This waterfall surges onward to join the larger body of water.

"Is that a river," I ask, "or a moving lake?"

River Woman smiles. "That's the Columbia River. Come on. We'll portage here. Some drops in the river, like our lives, are just too pre-cipitous to navigate. We'll take the trail down the mountain."

The trail is steep. I slip several times on loose gravel and struggle to catch my balance. I don't want to roll like a shattered snowball down the cliff.

We haul the boat down the serpentine cliff trail, then follow beside "our" river's path to the Columbia.

"This is a major artery," River Woman explains. "This river looks placid, but its currents are deceptively strong, powerful enough to divert an oil tanker from its path."

"Will our boat hold in these waters?" I'm more than a bit hesi-tant, eyeing our aluminum vessel and wooden paddles.

"Do we have a choice?"

"Yes, we could camp on the banks. . . at least for awhile."

River Woman stares hard at me. I meet her gaze, but flinch inside. I've come this far. I know the river reaches the sea. I sense that salty water woos River Woman more strongly than any other element in creation—water longing for itself, our own blood longing for its original mother.

I swallow hard and drop my pack into the canoe. River Woman grasps the gunnels, preparing to push us from shore.

I sit in the bow, spreading my feet wide. I want ballast to meet this current. My body feels diaphanous, like a leaf eddying without steerage along a stream.

Waves lap along the sides. We stay close to shore, but even here we are soon moving at tremendous speeds. The force of this water is too immense to resist.

I remember the stories of the Lewis and Clark expedition making this final passage along the Columbia to the sea. After years of hardship, hunger, and uncertainty, they shot through rapids that people native to the river portaged. The proximity of the sea magnetized them as no human lover ever could. The draw was deeper, more primal, more urgent than any short-lived tryst.

Now, moved by the same waters, I recognize the call of the sea. We move from freshwater into the first backwash of saltwater. The air changes, alive with ozone and a salty tang.

Late that afternoon, we pull the canoe onto a rocky shore. We set up camp, then hike across the dunes to the ocean shore.

I am too tired to comment. My arms and legs are weak and trembling, taxed beyond their capacity. In contrast, River Woman looks fresh, expectant.

"Watch the waves," she says.

I feel as well as see the power of the waves, sliding into land and then churning the shore's soft belly as it moves backward, tripping the next incoming wave.

"What is happening to the rocks, the driftwood, the sea-glass shards?"

"The waves are grinding them into sand," I reply without averting my gaze from the water.

"That's right, everything returning to its most fundamental elements. Molecules of water, mineral, air."

"This is death, isn't it River Woman? Everything unraveling to its simplest, first forms?"

"Yes," she says softly. "This is death, when the largest, widest current of your life reaches its end. The largest artery, the fullest experience, is your last."

I know in my bones that I'm too tired to fight that ending.

"We all work with the same elements, and shape them as we fancy." She seems to be talking more to herself than me. "Ultimately, though, the elements unravel. They slip off their form

*like an old overcoat, and return to their original, unmastered
selves."*

*The sun dips below the horizon and stars begin to appear in
the dusk.*

*"That's what I'm doing, too," I muse. "Returning to original
form. So simple, especially when you are tired."*

*My body offers no resistance as I settle into my sleeping bag on
the beach. I can already feel the night breeze and the dampness
unbraiding my bones. By morning I'll be sand on the beach.*

Reflections by Marlise Wabun Wind

*Marlise Wabun Wind is a mother, wife, home-schooler, and author of ten books
including* The Medicine Wheel *and* Woman of the Dawn. *She was a co-founder
of The Bear Tribe, a Native American Medicine Society based on the vision of Sun
Bear who was a Chippewa/Anishnabe teacher and medicine man. Wabun has
also been medicine helper to Sun Bear, a ceremonialist, a vision-quest guide, a
teacher of female and earth energy, and a lifetime seeker of how people can learn
to be the best human beings they can be.*

I went into menopause surgically. I had a hysterectomy when I was forty-
three or forty-four. For quite a number of years, including my last years at
the Bear Tribe, I had extremely heavy bleeding, and very, very painful periods
that were lasting longer and longer. After I left the Bear Tribe, my symptoms
worsened. I went to the doctor and was diagnosed with a large dermoid cyst.
The doctor wanted to do a complete hysterectomy then, but my husband,
Shawnodese, and I had both hoped we would have children, biologically.

So I refused the complete hysterectomy, had the dermoid-cyst surgery,
and spent a year trying to have a biological child, but continued to have
extreme problems with bleeding. When they did some scopes, they found I
had a very small carcinoma in situ. I weighed trying to have a biological
child against continuing to live, and continuing to live won. I had the complete hysterectomy. They took my womb apart and discovered a freckle-
sized cancerous area. They caught it at the very, very beginning. They
considered the hysterectomy a complete cure. It was.

Having the surgery was extremely difficult. I had a great deal of grief
over the hysterectomy and about having to give up the idea of ever having a

biological child.

I remember going into the surgery reading something from *Wildfire* magazine that Brooke Medicine Eagle had written about many women being called into the Grandmother Lodge early through hysterectomy because there was such a dearth of Grandmothers and Elders in that lodge. That gave me a great deal of comfort. I literally was reading the article going into surgery.

> . . . *many of us who are younger are being called into the Grandmother Lodge because there is an urgent need for the awakening of this function among women. Because of the crushing of the native cultures and the loss of the women's ways, there are few who sit in these Lodges and uphold the nurturing and renewing of the people. So younger, awakened ones of us are being called into the Lodge through many different means. Accept it as an honor.*[1]

I prayed a lot about the hysterectomy. I used the pipe during that time period. I think after the hysterectomy it's really important to allow yourself to grieve for losing a part of your body, and for losing a potential for one part of life. Most women who have hysterectomies have already had their children, and so they don't have that particular grief. But still you are losing the physical aspect of your womanhood. That doesn't mean you're losing your womanhood, and I think women often get confused on that point. In fact, I feel I am a lot more a woman than I was prior to that time, that I understand much more deeply what it means to be a woman.

Because I went through menopause surgically, I did go on hormone replacement therapy initially. My experience of Provera was just horrible. After about a month, I called it "the bitch hormone." I just stopped because I couldn't stand who I became when I took it. I did stay on estrogen because that was still the time when they were scaring you that if you went off it you would have a heart attack immediately. Eventually the estrogen didn't seem to be doing anything positive, and I stopped taking that, too. Occasionally I'll take an herbal phytoestrogen formula. I still have night sweats almost twenty years after the hysterectomy, but they don't bother me. I figure they're the estrogen surging through me. I think Brooke calls them "power surges" instead of hot flashes, and that always seemed like a good way to think of them.

It's good to know what's happening when you're having hot flashes, and to see if there's any pattern to them. If you can objectify them, and not say "it's a terrible experience," but rather look at what they're saying to *you,* I think that even if they don't go away, they don't bother you nearly as much. So I would recommend that to women.

The native people taught that as you went through menopause, you were able to see life in two ways. You had seen life as a woman who cycled, and now you could experience life as a man who did not cycle. You would have the ability, then, to pull from those two viewpoints and have them both for whatever you chose to look at. I think it gives you a much greater perspective when you've gone through menopause.

The cycling, the period, is such a large part of women's life. Hormones really do function in the body, and they change how you feel on a cyclical basis, which is good in some ways, but it's also very all-encompassing when it's going on. Any woman who's menstruating knows that. You gain a freedom of coming into yourself in a strong way when you are not cycling. You're not fighting the hormones to stay on an even keel.

When I look at young women coming into menarche, I see the effect that hormones have. I think, oh my goodness. I used to teach that how women see the world while they are on their period is maybe how the world really is, and everything else is a lie. When you are on your period, your energy is so large, and encompasses so much. But you also have very little ability to discriminate what comes out of your mouth, which is why women often get feisty and into fights when they are on their moon-time. You can put up with more when you are not on your period. When you are on your period, you can't ignore those things that you've been turning your eye away from the rest of the month. You want to bring them up, and you want to solve them. I don't think men ever experience life in quite that way. I think one of the sources of emotional depth that women have comes from the hormonal shifts we experience. When you no longer experience them, you certainly remember what it's like. But you're no longer driven by them.

I came out of the surgery and the recovery period realizing that I still wanted to have a child and almost immediately did all of the paperwork to be able to adopt. A friend of mine whom I had known at the Bear Tribe told me about a woman who ran an adoption agency who was open to spiritual people. I went to her, and we talked about what was most important to me, which was being able to come together with the child as early in its life as possible. At that point, Peru was the best place to be able to adopt children very early. I did all the paperwork, and nine months after I'd had the hysterectomy, I got the call that my daughter was available. If you know anything about adoptions, that is quite amazing. I thought that was very interesting that it was nine months after the surgery. I did not expect it to be anywhere near that soon. I also know I had lots of support from Bear Tribe people who were praying that the adoption go as smoothly as possible.

I went into the Mother Lodge and the Grandmother Lodge at about the same time. And then Sun Bear got sick. My daughter, Kyla, ended up traveling with me through Germany on one or two lecture tours that Sun Bear had been scheduled to do. She did a lot of world traveling with me when she was a little baby. I would not have done it without her, because I believe that the bonding between mother and child is absolutely critical.

When I was going into the Grandmother Lodge, I was taking on the responsibility of motherhood. I was keeping up with the responsibilities of being Sun Bear's medicine helper, and I was changing. It took a number of years for me to realize that the most important thing I could be doing was putting my energy into raising a child, in what I believe is the best way a child should be raised, which is with as much contact and love as possible. Eventually I just started giving up everything else and putting my energy into raising Kyla. I did have a mother's helper. I found after a time that I didn't want that. I had not gone through all the work of trying to have a child to have someone else raise the child. So I gave up my career because I wanted to be with my daughter.

Because I was an older mother, I think Kyla's experience has been very different. You know, when you're an older mother, you have a lot more patience. I think you have a lot more wisdom. Sometimes I feel like I'm her mother and grandmother at the same time. She keeps saying to me, "I can't wait for you to be grandma to my children, because I know you're going to be a wonderful grandma."

There were times when I was still doing the Bear Tribe work, and Kyla was with me in circles, and she would address me as "Grandmother." She knew that I was her mother, but she also knew that to other people I had become Grandmother.

I feel like I've been growing more into the name that Wallace Black Elk gave me many, many years ago in sweat lodge, *Inya Oyate*, which I'm told means "Mother of Nations." I've spent quite a number of years during the

Grandmother Lodge time doing what a lot of other women do in their younger years: experiencing life as a wife and mother. In many ways, it's been a very humbling experience for me because I have discovered how much time and energy it takes just to make relationships work well on a small level. I think in some ways it's easier to make relationships work on a grand level, when you don't have to be as intimate with people.

I've always wanted to find a better way for people to live together. Really the only way is to become that good householder that all spiritual traditions teach is the basis of true spirituality. But oftentimes people get so caught up in the grander part of spirituality that they don't spend enough time concentrating on what's close to home. We can't ever really change the world until we change the way we birth and raise children, because it's people that make the world.

When Kyla was a small child—and small children if they are loved are always very loving—when I would hold her, cuddle her, I would have a warmth in my solar plexus that I have never experienced with anything else—a sense of completeness, oneness with the world. The other time of course I've experienced it, and other people have, is with someone you love very greatly, when you feel at one. I also experienced that as a mother.

As we separate now, and I can feel that tie severing, there's a sense of loss, but also a sense of pride as I see that she is a woman now. A young woman who is capable of being her own person and will go into the world. I'm not sure what area she will choose, but whatever it is, she'll do wonderful things. And she's going to be a happy person, because she always has been. Part of that is nature. Her nature is to be happy. And part of that is that she's been raised in a way that we told her it was OK to stay that way.

It's going to feel like my heart's being ripped out when she actually goes to live away, but there's also pride that she's capable of doing that. And I know that once I heal my solar plexus ties, I will be ready to do some of the best work that I've ever done, in terms of writing and hopefully teaching again.

I remember learning that in some native traditions the grandmother and grandfather would raise the children, because the parents would be hunting and gathering. The grandparents who were not capable of doing that level of physical work would have the responsibility of the children. I think that must have been a wonderful thing in a culture where traditions did not change every decade, as they do in our society now. The mother and grandmother agreed on how the child should be raised. They worked together to raise the children.

For most women, when you come into the Grandmother Lodge, your responsibility is all the children. You have your own children, and now all the children are your children. Try to be as kind as you can be to the generation coming up. And try not to feed them—excuse me, I can't think of a better word—bullshit, because they know when they're being lied to. They respond by disbelief and sarcasm and rebellion, and eventually hatred of some sort or other.

We need to break down the worst old boys' network there is, saying that because my parents did this to me, it's OK for me to do this to my kids. We've got to stop mutilating children physically, emotionally, mentally, and spiritually. And we do that in all nations, whether they are "developing" or "developed," be it the female circumcision in Africa, or the male circumcision throughout the world, or our inability to stand the energy of our own children so that we throttle them or put them in car seats, or put them in front of the television set because we can't stand their spontaneous expression of life. And that's not to say there aren't times to have kids quiet down, but not to suppress their energy and teach them to be afraid of life coming through them on an energetic level.

There are a lot of little things women can do to help each other. When I see a mother doing a really good job of mothering in a situation, I go up and tell her. Or if I see children who are obviously loved and happy, tell the mother, "You're doing a wonderful job," because God knows, not enough people are telling her that. I think if more people in the Grandmother Lodge could do that, and support the younger women however they can, then it would make motherhood a more pleasant experience for a lot of people. You can feel so isolated, being a mother. That is so very, very difficult. It does take more than one person to give a child everything he or she needs.

Contact Marlise through either of the following websites: www.marlisewabun-wind.com or www.wabunwind.com.

CHAPTER NINE

NUTRITION for MENOPAUSAL WOMEN: BODY ENLIGHTENMENT

NUTRITION, THE FOOD WE TAKE INTO OUR BODIES, IS ONE OF THE PRIMARY ways we nurture our bodies. The better nourished our bodies are, the easier the transition through menopause. In the second section of the chapter, we will also be exploring ways of nourishing our spirit.

FOOD IS YOUR BEST SOURCE OF NUTRIENTS

You can supplement nutrients in three ways: with food, with a multivitamin and mineral supplement, and/or with single nutrients for specific deficiencies. Many patients ask if they should take nutritional supplements. Ultimately pills are a secondary, not a primary, source of nutrition.

Whole Food First

Your best source of nutrients is foods that are as close as possible to their natural state. Have you ever seen a Twinkie tree, a Danish pastry bush, or a Kool-Aid plant? The more refined and processed our food, the more nutrients we lose and the more health-defeating substances we gain, for example, preservatives, dyes, and chemical stabilizers. Preservatives are a boon for grocery stores but a hazard for our health. BHT, sodium nitrate, sodium nitrite, and other preservatives break down into noxious toxic substances in our bodies. Our health suffers; only our cadavers benefit.

Eating whole foods guarantees that we receive more nutrients and more fiber. Whole grains, for example, have far more nutrients and much more fiber than refined grains. Even extractor juicers, touted for their health-enhancing properties, can diminish the value of whole foods. A cup of extracted apple juice, for example, requires five fresh apples. The juice delivers a concentrated dose of sugar—yes, fructose or fruit sugar, but sugar nevertheless—and almost no fiber. You can easily drink a glass of apple juice, but could you eat five apples in one sitting? Not all juicers extract the fiber, however. Some (for example, the Vita-Mix) use the entire fruit or vegetable, including the nutrient- and fiber-rich pulp.

Organically Grown Foods Contain More Nutrients

According to California state law, "organic" means food grown without pesticides, insecticides, herbicides, or petroleum-based fertilizers. Certified organic farms have been "chemical-free" for at least three years. Recent studies demonstrate that organic foods have more nutrients than their conventionally grown counterparts.[1] Although organic foods may cost a bit more, they deliver more nutrients per serving, making up for the increased cost.

Macronutrients: Carbohydrates, Fats, and Water

Rather than focusing on isolated nutrients, the following discussion addresses three of the four major food groups, or "macronutrients": carbohydrates, fats, and water. In chapter 11, we will discuss the fourth major group, protein. If you make good choices in obtaining these four major nutrients, you will greatly increase your odds of ingesting the majority of the vitamins and minerals, or "micronutrients," you need as well.

COMPLEX CARBOHYDRATES REDUCE YOUR RISK FOR HEART DISEASE

Many popular diets recommend eating lots of protein and restricting carbohydrates as a way of boosting energy and promoting weight loss. Carbohydrates are blamed for increasing blood-sugar levels and thus fat production. What these diets overlook, however, is the difference between simple and complex carbohydrates.

Simple carbohydrates are refined grains and sugars, stripped of their fiber and many essential nutrients. I call them the "white wonders": white sugar, white flour, white rice, white bread, white pasta, and so on. The digestive tract quickly breaks down and absorbs these simple carbohydrates. Blood-sugar levels skyrocket, and the body converts any excess sugar into fats and cholesterol. Many "fat-free" foods are full of sugar, which quickly converts to fat in the body. If you want to reduce fat and cholesterol levels, avoid sugary foods!

Complex carbohydrates such as whole grains and beans contain lots of fiber, B vitamins and other nutrients. The digestive tract slowly absorbs high-fiber foods. This slow breakdown process helps stabilize blood-sugar levels and reduces insulin secretion. Insulin, a hormone produced in the pancreas, acts like a "key" to open cell walls so that blood sugar may enter. High blood-sugar levels stimulate increased insulin secretion. Fiber helps lower blood-sugar levels, which leads to reduced insulin production and lower body weight. Fiber also binds with cholesterol in the digestive tract, blocking cholesterol absorption.

Along with a high fat diet, high insulin levels and obesity increase your risk for heart disease. Recent studies demonstrate that the amount of fiber you eat more accurately predicts your risk of heart disease than saturated fat intake.[2,3] In other words, the more fiber you eat, the lower your risk for heart disease.

Complex carbohydrates also play a major role in increasing "satiety," the full sensation in your stomach that signals you have had enough to eat. Because complex carbohydrates contain more fiber, they provide more bulk in the stomach and make the stomach feel "full" with fewer calories. A cup of French fries and three cups of brown rice contain approximately the same number of calories. You can easily eat a cup of French fries at a meal, but could you comfortably eat three cups of cooked brown rice at one sitting?

Eating the Standard American Diet (SAD), most Americans consume only 9 grams of fiber per day. The American Dietetic Association recommends eating 25 to 35 grams of fiber daily. Including more complex carbohydrates in your diet can help reduce weight, insulin and blood sugar levels while providing the body with a healthy source of fuel and nutrients. As a bonus, these high-fiber foods can also reduce your risk of heart disease.

Digesting Carbohydrates

Our saliva contains several important enzymes that begin the process of carbohydrate digestion. Normally saliva is slightly acidic, ranging from pH 6.6 to 6.8. If salivary pH strays from this normal range, the digestive enzymes no longer function properly, and we may have difficulty digesting carbohydrates. Food allergies or sensitivities may also thwart carbohydrate digestion.

Simple carbohydrates: White sugar, brown sugar, succanat (raw sugar), molasses, corn syrup, dextrose, corn starch, white flour, white pasta, white rice, white bread, white flour tortillas, white flour bakery products (muffins, English muffins, cookies, cakes, and so on).

Complex carbohydrates: Brown rice, millet, barley, whole wheat, rye, oats, quinoa, pinto beans, black beans, red beans, lentils, whole wheat bread.

Wheat, corn, and soybeans, for example, are some of the most common food allergens in North America. If you have difficulty digesting carbohydrates, consider checking your salivary pH and/or testing for food allergies.

DIET AND THE GLYCEMIC INDEX

Many of us know the effects of sweets and junk food. Few are aware, however, that certain "healthy" foods can also dramatically increase blood-sugar levels. The "glycemic index" measures how quickly the carbohydrate in a food enters the bloodstream as blood sugar. Not all carbohydrates were created equal! Those foods with a high glycemic index cause a quick increase in blood-sugar levels, while low glycemic index foods help maintain lower, steadier blood-sugar levels. Beans, for example, have a low glycemic index, helping to maintain steady blood-sugar levels over several hours.

A food's ability to increase blood sugar is not always directly related to the number of calories. Carrots, although low in calories, cause a sharp rise in blood-sugar levels.

To help stabilize blood-sugar levels

♦ Choose foods that are low on the glycemic index.

♦ Eat five or six smaller meals for a steadier "burn" of energy.

♦ Eat beans to help stabilize blood-sugar levels for up to four hours.

♦ Emphasize complex carbohydrates (whole grains and beans) and avoid simple carbohydrates (white flour products, white sugar, refined grains).

♦ Choose high-fiber foods to help steady blood-sugar levels.

High glycemic index foods (eliminate these or combine them with low glycemic index foods): corn flakes, carrots, maltose, honey, potatoes, white rice.

Medium glycemic index foods: buckwheat, sweet corn, sweet potatoes and yams, oranges, porridge oats, brown rice.

Low glycemic index foods (emphasize these): black-eyed peas, chickpeas, apples, kidney beans, lentils, soybeans, peanuts, milk and milk products

---

ESSENTIAL FATTY ACIDS

Despite its maligned media image, fat is a vital nutrient. Cholesterol, for example, is the building block for all our reproductive hormones, and every cell wall in the body is made of cholesterol and fatty acids.

Our bodies can manufacture several types of fat and cholesterol from other substances, but two fats cannot be produced inside the body: linoleic acid and alpha-linolenic acid. These are referred to as "essential fatty acids" because our body cannot manufacture them, yet they are essential for normal, healthy bodies. We must consume these essential nutrients in our diet.

What's the Difference between Fats and Oils?

The main difference between fats and oils is the number of double bonds or "links" in their chains, and how solid or fluid they are at room temperature. Fats and oils are made of long chains of carbons with hydrogen atoms attached. Think of them as long trains, with each carbon representing a boxcar on the train.

Imagine the "hitches" between the boxcars as single or double connections, or "bonds" to use chemistry terms. The fewer the double hitches between the boxcars, the more solid the fat is at room temperature. Fats have only single "hitches" between the carbon atoms, which explains why they are solid at room temperature.

At the double hitches or "bonds," the carbon atoms are loosely attached to each other. Johanna Budwig, MD, describes a double hitch on the chain as ". . .fragile there, loose; it absorbs water easily—as if you were to fray a smooth silk thread in one place and then draw it through water. The frayed part absorbs water, or dye, more easily. In the same way, these fatty acid chains with their weak, unsaturated connections, form protein associations very easily. **The fatty acids become water soluble through this association with protein.**"[emphasis added][4]

Blood is a watery substance, and oil and water usually do not mix. Unsaturated fats, however, can become water soluble through their association with protein. The unsaturated fats, with numerous "double hitches" to use the train analogy above, can "mix" with the watery blood when eaten with protein-rich foods. Because unsaturated fats can "dissolve" in the blood, they can move through the blood and nourish appropriate cells.

In contrast, saturated fats cannot dissolve in the watery fluid of the blood. Hydrogenated oils are also insoluble in water. These solid fats "separate" in the blood, like oil and vinegar in salad dressing. Insoluble solid fats, such as all animal fats, cannot circulate through the network of fine capillaries in the body; instead, they deposit along larger blood vessels walls, compromising circulation and promoting heart disease.

Quality Is as Important as Quantity

Most margarine is made with altered fats called "trans-fatty acids." *Cis* and *trans* formations describe the three-dimensional structure of a molecule. Normally the hydrogen atoms attached to carbon in a fat molecule are on the same "side" of the molecule (*cis* formation). Think of the train with hydrogen atoms attached to the same side of the boxcar. Heating oil and adding hydrogen atoms changes the molecular structure. These altered *trans*- fatty acids have hydrogen molecules attached on opposite sides of the molecule, across from ("trans") each other.

Only now are we beginning to understand the long-term effects of consuming these altered trans-fatty acids. Women eating a diet high in trans-fatty acids (for example, margarine, vegetable shortening, and fried foods) have a much higher risk of developing coronary heart disease.[5] In contrast, people eating a "Mediterranean" diet—high in fresh vegetables, fruits, fish, and olive oil—have significantly lower risk of heart disease.[6]

How Much Fat Do I Need in My Diet?

Usually dietary recommendations suggest the percentage of calories derived from fat rather than a specific amount. For people consuming a traditional Asian diet, about 10 percent of their calories come from fat. In contrast, most North Americans derive a prodigious 40 to 50 percent of their calories from fat!

Aim for a diet with 10 to 15 percent of your calories derived from fats. Ideally those fats would be naturally occurring oils in the food you eat, supplemented with olive oil for cooking and small amounts of flax, hemp or other cold-pressed oils for salad dressings. Eliminate saturated fats and hydrogenated oils.

HEALING WATERS: ARE YOU DEHYDRATED?

Certain foods have a diuretic effect, causing water loss, while others encourage the body to hold water, leading to bloating and water retention. One cup of a caffeinated beverage, for example, causes a loss of two cups of fluid.

Alcohol also acts as a diuretic in the body. After overindulging, dehydration contributes to the characteristic "hangover."

In April 1990, *Business Magazine* in Canada reported that millions of North Americans consume two-thirds of their water from coffee. Several million more imbibe one-third or more of their water in the form of beer. That means that by the end of the day, most North Americans have a water deficit.

Not drinking enough fluid ironically may cause water retention. Decreased fluid means increased breakdown products, or "toxins," that the body cannot eliminate through the kidneys, so the body holds water to try to dilute these toxic products. The buildup of metabolic waste products can lead to fatigue, foggy thinking, irritability, headaches, joint and muscle pain, and a host of other symptoms.

Water Quality

Most municipalities add chlorine to drinking water to kill bacteria and other organisms. Chlorine serves an important function in delivering water to our homes; however, ingesting chlorine destroys many nutrients, particularly the B vitamins, and increases xenoestrogen activity in the body. *Xeno* means foreign, so "xenoestrogens" are foreign substances with estrogen-like activity that contribute to estrogen dominance.

Plastics can release chemicals that have xenoestrogen effects in the body. Drinking water stored in plastic bottles may contain chemicals that have migrated into the water, especially if the plastic container is heated. Plastic water pipes, particularly those made of PVC, can leach chemicals into the water.

Check the bottom of your plastic bottles. One form of plastic, marked with the number seven, is much more stable and less likely to migrate into the water. Many health-food stores now carry half-gallon water containers made with number-seven plastic. Although not the safest for transport, glass is the most stable form of water bottle.

Nutrition and the Menopausal Passage

The better nourished you are during this time in your life, the easier the menopausal transition will be. This chapter offers basic information to help you make healthy dietary choices. Ideally you would work with a health-care provider trained in dietary nutrition (not just supplements) who can help tailor dietary suggestions for your particular needs.

FASTING: BODY ENLIGHTENMENT

Appropriate cleansing and fasting can help prepare the body for the menopausal passage. I'm not talking about obsessively "cleaning out" the "dirty" colon, but rather offering the body an opportunity to discard unnecessary wastes. The smaller the backlog of wastes and toxins, the easier the hormonal transitions can be during perimenopause.

Most of us approach fasting and cleansing with gritted teeth. We focus on hunger, discomfort, and deprivation. I don't mean to belittle these symptoms, rather I want to expand the range of possibilities for what this internal "housecleaning" can bring into our lives.

First, let's differentiate between fasting and cleansing. Fasting means the complete absence of a particular substance or activity. Most of us think of abstaining from food, but a fast could include eliminating water, conversation, sex, and/or media exposure (TV, newspaper, radio, and so on).

Cleansing focuses on clearing waste from the body. Many companies now offer "cleanse" programs that are simply supplements added to your usual diet. The supplements usually include several "cathartic" herbs that promote bowel movements by irritating the colon (for example, senna, cascara sagrada, and buckthorn bark). In addition, the "cleanse" programs usually include dietary fiber (such as psyllium seed husks); and/or bentonite clay, to remove candida die-off, parasites, and mucous from the intestines.

The cathartic herbs are only meant for short-term use, no longer than a month at a time. Initially the cathartic herbs do increase bowel movements by irritating the intestinal muscles and thereby increasing "peristalsis," the wavelike movement of the digestive system muscles that eventually causes a bowel movement. Too much stimulation, however, can cause intestinal cramping. Even worse, after several months of use, the intestinal muscles stop reacting to the irritation and do not move at all! Taking prescription medications for constipation have the same effect (that is, *no* effect) with long-term use.

Recent studies also demonstrate that using the cathartic herbs for a year or more causes "intestinal melanosis," a condition of increased melanin production in the colon. Melanosis may be a precursor to colon cancer. The bottom line: find other ways than the cathartic herbs for keeping your bowel movements regular.

Cleansing Safely and Effectively

Most cleanse programs offer one-size-fits all instructions without regard for your particular body's ability to remove wastes. Pushing the body too far, too fast can cause more harm than good. You need a reliable method to determine the waste-removal pace your body can safely sustain.

If you want to pursue a cleanse program, I would encourage you to test saliva and urine pH before beginning. Saliva and urine pH reflect the balance of "electrolytes" in the body. Electrolytes are minerals, such as calcium, sodium, magnesium, and chlorine. Hence, pH is a reflection of electrolytes, which is a reflection of mineral levels in the body.

The minerals are vital components in the waste-removal processes in the body. If the mineral/electrolyte levels are too high or too low, the body cannot successfully remove waste. Depending on the cleanse program you are following, the body may dump a lot of waste material. If the body does not have adequate electrolyte levels to remove the waste, it will be reabsorbed. The body gains nothing from the arduous cleanse process if you are unable to clear the waste material.

The Arise and Shine program was the first to incorporate pH testing. For more information, visit www.ariseandshine.com or call (800) 688-2444.

Fasting for Physical Health

I was seventeen years old the first time I completed a three-day water fast. I found instructions in a booklet at the health-food store. Thankfully the program was well constructed. I drank lemon water and took alfalfa tablets, which are a good source of minerals and fiber (remember the importance of minerals, electrolytes, and pH levels). With my history of childhood illnesses and dozens of rounds of antibiotics, my body was extremely toxic, even at that young age. Even though I had eaten well and had been running regularly for four years, I experienced many detoxification symptoms during the fast (foggy thinking, fatigue, headaches, joint aches, and muscle weakness).

One of the greatest gifts of that particular fast was learning a healthy way of reintroducing food. Correctly introducing food after a fast enhances the effects of fast. Eating the wrong foods, or introducing them in the incorrect order, can undo all of your hard work.

After a water fast, introduce food in the following order:

- Day 1, breaking the fast: Drink diluted fruit or vegetable juices (half water, half juice). Sip a couple of tablespoons of juice every 15 to 20 minutes throughout the day.

- Days 2 and 3, after the fast: Add fresh fruits (or, if you do not eat fruits, raw vegetables).

- Days 3 and 4: Add lightly steamed vegetables.

- Days 5 and 6: Add grains and bread.

- Days 7 and 8: Add dairy products.

- Days 9 and10: Add meats, fish, and beans.

Fasting and Weight Loss

Many people fast for weight loss. In the long run, fasting is a poor method for shedding extra pounds. Yes, you may drop pounds during the actual fast. With a sudden, major drop in calorie intake, however, the body slows its metabolic rate to a crawl. The body perceives that it is under siege and slows to survive what it perceives to be a period of famine.

When you reintroduce foods, the body quickly replaces any lost weight *plus* a few pounds. The body wants "insurance" weight to make sure that it can survive another period of deprivation in the future.

Another potential danger of fasting for weight loss is the mental attitude some people develop. In an extreme, fasting can lead to anorexia. Food becomes the "enemy," the source of our body-image woes. For someone who is out of control, food becomes one of the few things they can master. Overcontrol leads to a twisted relationship with food.

We live in a culture of extremes. North America has one of the highest obesity rates in the world. Simultaneously we have many people, especially women, who suffer with eating disorders. They are literally starving themselves in a sea of plenty.

Fasting can be approached as another form of control or deprivation. At its best and healthiest, however, fasting can eliminate distraction and clear space for Creator's presence in our lives.

Making Way for the Divine

My next major experience of fasting was at age twenty-two, when I completed a four-day vision quest with an Anishnabe (Chippewa) elder. Many native peoples have a vision-quest tradition; there is no one right or wrong way to complete a vision quest. In this case, the fast is not so much for renewal of the body as for consecration of the soul. The absence of food, conversation, and human stimulation makes space for the Divine to enter our lives.

Up to that point in my life, my mind had ruled my conscious activity. According to a friend, I had a Ferrari mind in a Fiat body. I could outdistance almost any mental challenger in about three seconds flat.

During the first day of the vision quest, alone in a four-foot diameter circle on the edge of the mountain, I struggled to simply stay seated. I reviewed all of my major life relationships, relived every hurt and trauma, and generally charged up and down any mental slope that would distract me from my present circumstance. Gradually over the next three days, my mind quieted, until finally no thoughts circulated in my mind. For the first time in my life, my mind was quietly at peace.

In this silence, I began to "hear" all of the elements of creation around me. The trees, rocks, and animals all had volumes to speak. I could hear those elements of creation only when my own motor-mind had finally stilled. Fasting made way for silence, which in turn made space for wisdom to enter my heart-mind, a much deeper and wiser aspect of myself than the conscious mind that helped me navigate in my daily life.

I have continued to seek solitude and silence at every major decision point in my life. I have sought isolated beaches, wilderness trails, mountaintops, and even a burial cairn in the north of Scotland. I emerge from the "deprivation" of food, water, and human companionship with a fullness of spirit.

Fasting from Speaking

I have also experienced "fasting" in groups, in silent meditation retreats. Although the retreats included food and water, the abstinence from speaking brought a profound inner clarity. I recognized how much energy I spent in speaking. The longer the period of silence, the more power my words had when I began to speak again.

I also began to realize how much mental activity I expended worrying about other people's thoughts and attitudes. During one silent retreat at

Breitenbush, a hot-springs community nestled in the mountains of Oregon, I climbed into one of the hot-spring tubs after dinner. I settled into the steaming water, and leaned my head back to watch snow sifting from the night sky. Three other people were already relaxing in the tub. We settled into the waters without comment. As I emerged from the tub, I suddenly realized I had chosen a spot without the usual mental machinations that accompany any social situation: "I wonder if I will disturb them? Is there room for me here? Will the people be welcoming? What if I'm uncomfortable with the people, the conversation? Will they be offended if I leave?"

I saw how much mental energy I usually expended just in the simple act of choosing a spot to soak. Those mental machinations only became apparent when they were absent. The outer silence made way for inner silence. By discarding extraneous conversation, I was able to still the inner chatter that drained so much energy.

Weekly Fasts

If you are interested in fasting as a way of supporting your spiritual and physical development, consider adopting the rhythm of a weekly fast.

For ten years, I fasted every Sunday. The exact form evolved over the years. Initially I drank only water and continued my daily routine. As I learned more about liver function and pH levels, I drank whole fruit and vegetable juices during the day. Even later, I discovered the importance of adding an enema at the end of the day or the next morning to assist the body in moving drier stools.

You may choose to fast from food, water, and/or conversation. Phyllis Rodin, who has devoted her life to peace and human evolution, spends every Friday in silence. These weekly immersions in silence have kept her inner "batteries" charged for years.

The following are suggestions for developing your own fasting routine. Focus on ways of making space for the Divine, like clutter-clearing for the soul. Remove distractions and choose activities that deeply nourish your body, mind, and soul.

- ♦ Choose a natural setting or a quiet space where you will not be disturbed. Wilderness areas innately have more "qi" or life force and can support the restoration of your own body's vitality. Even in the midst of a major city, though, you can create a peaceful sanctuary.

- Decide what your fast will include: food, water, conversation, media, sex

- Focus on deep intimacy with yourself. You might choose mediation, music, or self-massage with essential oils diluted in pure vegetable oil to lavish on yourself. Practice the sacred art of indulgence. Remember, you are wooing the Divine.

- Make space for creativity, for example, writing, painting, singing, and/or dancing. Often you will have much clearer insight during your fasting day.

- Drink plenty of diluted juice and herb teas. You may need to eat steamed vegetables and small amounts of protein.

If you are hypoglycemic or have special health needs, consult with a health-care provider experienced in fasting to modify your program. You may benefit most from a media/conversation fast rather than from a food fast.

Reflections by the Reverend Dr. Julia Turner

Born in the Netherlands, Julia studied at The Royal Conservatory in the Hague. She has completed advanced studies in philosophy, psychology, religion, operations research and mathematics, music mythology and brain-mind technologies at European and United States universities. This combination of disciplines has lead to pioneering work on living alchemy, the art of evolutionary transformation. In her workshops, she teaches multiple modalities such as brain-mind technologies, music, movement, high-powered visualization, critical-thinking skills, and inner- directed discipline to empower the process of becoming the authentic Self. She is the founder of the Academy of Holistic Arts and Sciences.

I'm Dutch, and Dutch people generally don't make a big deal about anything. For me, menopause was a nonevent. Menopause is a natural state, a part of life.

My children leaving for college was a much bigger event. I was so caught up in my role as a mother and taking care of my children that for a couple of months I kept buying stuff for the kids. I'd forgotten to ask myself, "What do *I* actually like?" So by the time menopause came around, I had come through that particular phase, and I knew pretty well what I liked and what I didn't like.

One thing has shifted tremendously, actually. I will not allow other people to waste my time. If something is uninteresting, or people are wasting my time, then I say, "No, I'm sorry, I'm not going to do that because in these next thirty or forty years I have, I'm going to create my masterpiece, with everything that I've done before."

The women I know who are in their fifties, who have just gone through or are going through menopause, are incredibly competent women. They have worked very, very hard. They have neglected themselves tremendously. They are caught up in survival mode because of the financial turmoil created by the Enron phenomenon and the telecommunication collapse. These women thought they had some money. Suddenly they have nothing and have to start all over again. I have had to face the very same issues.

Everyone in our generation has Pluto in Leo, the call for creative self-realization. We are the "flower power" children, who started coloring outside the lines. Many of us forgot about the need to self-actualize, and instead shifted into the career mode and the doing mode. Suddenly it's collapsing all around us. Now we have to rebuild, first during menopause, which in this country is advertised as a disease, which it is *not*. It's a natural physiological process. Second, most of us are fat because we're so overstressed that our adrenals have stopped working. We don't have to do that. Third, we cannot continue in the old mode. We need to color outside the box.

No, we are not going to play golf in Florida. After having raised our children, we are going to explore our creative side. Now if we combine all that we've learned—including from our career—with our creativity, we can cook everything together into a profitable, successful vocation that is self-supporting.

In order to create this new vocation, you have to take care of your mind and your physical body. You take care of your mind through meditation and prayer, however you want to do it. You take care of your mind through breathing techniques. And you take care of your physical body through qigong, yoga, and some weight lifting to prevent osteoporosis. Lifting weights on an empty stomach and eating protein thirty minutes later will activate human growth hormone. You can even reverse osteoporosis.

Anybody who starts a spiritual path and does a lot of spiritual work first learns how to use the breath to control emotions, because those are left-brain belief structures and left-brain constructs; they are reactionary. So breath is the first thing you learn to control. I have a support system of a daily program of breathing, qigong, and yoga that also supports physical and emotional balance. For anyone having problems with menopause, working with the breath can help tremendously

Eating good foods is so important. And that's not your ordinary American diet, by a long shot. I know to eat more black beans to avoid hot flashes, and to eat cabbage soups for the indole-3-carbinole, a phytoestrogen. Pomegranates are very good for the ovaries; they contain tiny amounts of estrone.

I have a three-horsepower blender. I crunch up a lot of vegetables and a lot of seeds. That's really very powerful. You stay wrinkle free, which is a nice aspect to it. But you also stay disease free. You make your body alkaline. That's very useful.

Give yourself the time to exercise. Create that. Demand that. A healthy body is the underlying structure for creating the next exciting phase of your life.

Create some sort of a sabbatical; step back for a while. You don't have to take off a full year. A guided retreat would be very useful, but not because you have to improve yourself. Self-help books don't work because they always make you wrong. You're never good enough. It's the tyranny of potential. Self-improvement is not the key.

Transforming into more of who you are is very, very important. Allow everything that has been stuffed away for so long to re-emerge. That transformation needs to be supported in a very creative, fun way.

Creating a whole new state of being, thinking outside the box, and embracing your true self and your true nature, and also making it work financially, requires paying attention to practical things. That's where the New Age has missed the mark: "Do what you love and the money will follow." No, you need to have a structure, and some practical tools. Look at your weaknesses, strengthen those, or find a way around them by having somebody else do that for you. Spirituality also has a very pragmatic part; it ends in action. Real spirituality, any kind of spiritual or mystical path, is always laced with true action. You have to follow through, you have to do it. And there will be moments of great discomfort that are not fun at all.

You have to view situations from a higher perspective and keep asking the question, "What is the lesson in this? What is this about?" Not why, forget about why. Why is a boring question. What is this about? What is the lesson in this? How can I find a solution? There's a problem, there's a cause, and the solution always lies within the problem itself.

Just like mathematics, you have to shift your consciousness to see the solution. You move to a higher progression in order to solve the problem. Staying within the same way of thinking will not work. You need to shift your perspective. You might do that with a coach, a spiritual counselor, or a mentor. You may also choose to gather a group of women who are going through the same thing. Create enough trust to brainstorm. Support each other in taking action and following through.

So many menopausal women are also going through divorces and losses. This can be a very difficult time for women. We have to redefine how it's going to be, moving away from the crone and creating a new paradigm.

Before you become the crone, spend thirty years discovering your creative self. Find your unique treasure, become totally comfortable with it, and then give that creative gift for the good of all, in service of the world. This concept does not exist in the Western culture. I offer this new understanding of creativity as service as a gift to other women. The "service" I'm describing is not about being Mother Teresa. It's about finding your unique talent, exploring it, practicing it, and then expressing it in the world.

So, in other words, forget about retiring. Just recreate yourself. One phase is over. Now let's recreate it, let's do it differently than it has been done before, and get on with it.

You may contact her at drjuliaturner@yahoo.com or (703) 938-2465.

CHAPTER TEN

EXERCISE for MENOPAUSAL WOMEN: MEDITATION in MOTION

DESPITE THE JOGGING CRAZE OF THE EIGHTIES AND THE AEROBICS FAD OF the nineties, less than 20 percent of the U.S. population exercises regularly.

THE BENEFITS OF EXERCISE

Why should you bother to leave the comfort of your sofa or office chair? Review the health goals you set for yourself earlier (see chapter 2). Are you still interested in fulfilling your vision of health? If the answer is "Yes," carefully consider how exercise may assist you in achieving your goals.

Banish Hot Flashes

Exercise can be a powerful ally during menopause. Women who exercise aerobically at least 3.5 hours a week have about 75 percent fewer hot flashes.[1] Those 3.5 hours of exercise are spread over the course of a week, approximately 30 minutes per day, not 3.5 hours all at once.

Lower Blood Pressure

Women with mild to moderate hypertension may be able to control blood pressure with exercise alone. A group of postmenopausal women began an exercise program of walking thirty minutes, three or four times a week. After three weeks, they increased their walking speed and extended the time to forty to forty-five minutes per session. After twelve weeks, the women's aerobic fitness level was unchanged, but resting and submaximal exercise blood pressure dropped significantly, meaning their blood pressure did not elevate as much during exercise. Both systolic and diastolic blood pressure readings (the upper and lower numbers) dropped over the course of the twelve-week exercise training.[2]

More postmenopausal women die of coronary heart disease than other condition (including breast cancer), so this study offers great news. Even walking, a low-intensity aerobic exercise, can have profound effects on cardiovascular health.

Boost Your Immune System

Did you know that a daily walk strengthens your immune system as well as your heart? Moderate exercise increases white blood-cell activity, particularly the neutrophils, white blood cells that fight viral infections.[3, 4] Excessive training, however, can reduce neutrophil activity and may decrease resistance to infections.[5] Natural killer cells, important defense cells also linked with cancer prevention, increase after moderate exercise sessions.

Just as our body has a normal "physiological window" for hormones, we also have a normal range for exercise. Too little exercise will not stimulate immune cells, yet too much exercise may deplete the immune system. Aim for the amount of exercise that is "just right" for your particular body to boost the health of your immune system.

One martial arts master used to instruct his students to give only 80 percent of their energy in a training session. "If you give 100 percent," he would say, "you have nothing left in reserve." Exercising at 70 to 80 percent of your capacity means that you have a bit left over to accrue interest in your energy bank account. Most Westerners have no concept of nurturing a reserve of energy. We spend what we have and then some. Especially when you are beginning an exercise program, do only 70 to 80 percent of what you think you can. If you are certain you could walk for twenty minutes, for example, walk for fifteen.

Stabilize Blood-Sugar Levels

We discussed earlier how processed "white" foods enter the bloodstream like lightening, causing blood sugar to skyrocket and then crash. In those suffering with noninsulin-dependent diabetes, insulin receptor sites become resistant to insulin. Receptor sites are like baseball gloves that catch a specific substance. Once bonded with the baseball glove, the substance catalyzes certain activities in the cell. "Resistant" receptor sites do not allow the substance to bond. In essence, the catcher's mitt is closed. When insulin bonds with an insulin receptor site, it acts like a "key," opening the "lock" on a cell wall so that blood sugar can enter. Diabetics have high blood-sugar levels, but the glucose cannot move into the cells until insulin unlocks the "door."

Exercise makes insulin receptor sites more receptive so that insulin can bond and "unlock" the cell wall, allowing glucose to enter. Blood-sugar levels normalize because glucose is moving into the cells instead of remaining in the bloodstream. Exercise also stabilizes blood-sugar levels by affecting the basal metabolic rate (BMR), the speed at which our bodies "burn" energy. After exercising, the BMR remains elevated for up to six hours, which means our bodies burn more calories during that time. As we age, the BMR tends to decline, but exercise can reverse that trend.[6]

Additional Benefits

Exercise supports your body in many other ways too; it improves sleep, reduces stress and anxiety, and increases bone-mineral density. In chapter 9, we discussed how exercise can benefit bone health.

Components of a Balanced Exercise Program

Rather than repeating one form of movement over and over again, our bodies thrive on a variety of activities. Often exercise programs will focus on only one type of exercise, such as endurance training or stretching. Ideally a balanced program would incorporate endurance, strength building, stretching, and coordination exercise throughout the week. You may not be able to include all of the activities every day, but you can aim to incorporate each type of movement several times over the course of a week.

ENDURANCE EXERCISE

Endurance measures the body's ability to exercise for an extended period of time. The best endurance-building exercise is aerobic activity. Any rhythmic movement that increases heart rate, deepens breathing, and uses the large muscles of the leg qualifies as aerobic exercise. Sudden stop-start activities, such as tennis or volleyball, do not qualify as "aerobic" because they do not maintain the steady, rhythmic pace of aerobic exercises such as walking, swimming, and running.

The "FIT" (Frequency, Intensity, Time) concept outlines the minimum amount of exercise you need to improve aerobic fitness. If you want to improve cardiovascular fitness, you need to increase these parameters gradually over time:

Frequency

In order to develop cardiovascular fitness, you need to exercise aerobically at least three times a week.

Intensity Refers to how intensely you are working the heart. For beginners, the "target heart rate," or recommended intensity, is 60 to 70 percent of maximum heart rate. (See below for how to calculate your maximum and target heart rates.).

Timing Your aerobic workout should last at least fifteen to twenty minutes. Fitness experts used to think aerobic activity had to be continuous. Now we are learning that aerobic exercise scattered throughout the day has as much benefit as one concentrated aerobic session. The combination of a ten-minute walk with the dog before work, five minutes of climbing stairs during lunch, and another walk with the dog when you get home still qualifies as twenty minutes of aerobic exercise.[7]

Length You need to exercise regularly for at least six weeks before you can measure physiological improvements (for example, increased heart and lung efficiency). Of course you don't have to wait six weeks to notice lots of other improvements such as deeper sleep, brighter moods, and increased agility.

MAXIMUM AND TARGET HEART RATES

Maximum heart rate marks the maximum number of beats per minute your heart can safely endure. Pushing beyond the maximum heart rate may damage your heart. To figure your maximum heart rate, subtract your age from 220:

220 - _____ (your age) = _____ beats per minute (maximum heart rate)

Example of maximum heart rate: Elizabeth is fifty-seven years old. Her maximum heart rate is 220 - 57 = 163 beats per minute.

At your target heart rate, you should still be able to talk while exercising. When exercising at your target heart rate, you receive all the benefits of exercise without straining the heart. To calculate your target heart rate, see the formula below.

The resting heart rate is the number of times your heart beats in one minute when you are relaxed. You can count your pulse easily at the neck. Place your forefinger flat against your neck with the tip pointed upward toward your chin. Slide your finger to the side, into the trough on either side of your throat, and you easily will feel your pulse. Rest your finger lightly against your neck—you don't need to press hard to feel the pulse.

[(220 - your age _____) - resting heart rate _____] x .65 + resting heart rate _____ = target heart rate.

Example of target heart rate: Mary is 52 years old, and her resting heart rate is 72. Begin by subtracting her age from 220 (to calculate maximum heart rate): 220 - 52 = 168. Now subtract her resting heart rate: 168 - 72 = 96. Multiply by .65 (96 x .65 = 62). Finally, add back in the resting heart rate: 62 + 72 = 134 = target heart rate.

For advanced exercisers and athletes, aim for 75 to 85 percent of your maximum heart rate. Use the above formula, but multiply by .75 or .85 instead of .65.

CHARACTERISTICS OF AEROBIC EXERCISE:

- ◆ Rhythmic and continuous

- ◆ Uses the large muscles of the body (legs)

- ◆ ncreases heart rate to target heart rate

- ◆ Deepens breathing

Types of aerobic exercise:

- ◆ Walking
- ◆ Jogging or running
- ◆ Swimming
- ◆ Hiking
- ◆ Bicycling
- ◆ Rowing
- ◆ Backpacking
- ◆ Stair climbing

Types of nonaerobic exercise

These nonaerobic exercises develop other important aspects—for example, eye-hand coordination or strength—but they do not qualify as aerobic exercise.

- ◆ Tennis
- ◆ Basketball
- ◆ Volleyball
- ◆ Baseball
- ◆ Weight lifting
- ◆ Water skiing
- ◆ Wind surfing
- ◆ Horseback riding (the horse gets the aerobic points!)

STRENGTH-BUILDING EXERCISE

Strength-building exercise increases the muscles' ability to exert force against resistance, for example, lifting an object or throwing a ball. Over time, strength-building exercise increases muscle size. Because men have higher testosterone levels, they develop larger muscles more quickly. Women, in contrast, increase muscle strength by 44 percent before their muscles increase in size. For women, strong muscles do not necessarily mean large muscles.

When asked the single most important factor to slow aging in the body, researcher William Evans immediately responded, "Lift weights." Each year after age thirty-five, our bodies gain one and a half pounds of fat and lose a half-pound of muscle. Our scales measure the increase in fat but cannot detect the loss of muscle, which affects both our body shape and our metabolism.

At rest, one pound of fat burns approximately two calories a day. In comparison, a pound of muscle burns thirty-four calories a day! Losing muscle and gaining fat means that our bodies burn fewer calories per day. As our metabolism slows, we convert more of our food calories into fat. We enter a vicious cycle: more fat means fewer calories burned means more food calories converted into fat. No wonder we have more trouble maintaining a normal weight after age thirty-five!

Strength-building exercise can prevent that half-pound per year muscle loss. You are never too old to begin. Even elderly nursing home residents (ages eighty-six to ninety-six) significantly benefited from a weight-training program.[8] With gradual training, you can even increase muscle mass.

Research in the early 1990s demonstrated that exercise programs combining aerobic and resistance exercise catalyzed three times more fat loss than aerobic exercise alone. Knowing how many more calories muscles burn at rest, you can understand why resistance exercises, for example, weight lifting, would increase fat loss.[9]

CALORIES BURNED AT REST	MUSCLE	FAT
AMOUNT LOST AFTER AGE 35	34 calories/pound/day	2 calories/pound/day
AMOUNT GAINED AFTER AGE 35	0.5 pound/year (sedentary)	1.5 pounds per year (sedentary)

FLEXIBILITY

Stretching exercise increases the suppleness of joints and muscle tissue. Stretching lubricates joints, increases blood flow in the muscles, and improves flexibility. Lack of flexibility can increase muscle soreness and heighten the chance of muscle injury.

In addition to feeling good, stretching encourages proper muscle repair. Stretching reminds muscle tissue of its normal movement pattern so that the muscle fibers repair in the right direction. Without stretching, an injured muscle protects itself by laying down a tangled mass of connective tissue. This scar tissue can disrupt a muscle's normal movement, leading to pain and reduced range of motion.

As with any type of exercise, our bodies have an optimal range for stretching. Both too little and too much stretching can cause muscles and connective tissue to shrink. What is the right amount? Aim for at least five minutes of stretching per day. As we age, stretching becomes an increasingly important part of our exercise routine to keep muscles and joints supple.

In addition to stretching, our bodies need "range-of-motion" (ROM) exercises, meaning activities that take a joint through its full scope of movement. The shoulder, for example, can extend forward, above, and backward; reach to the side; and rotate in a circle. The wrist can flex forward and to the side, extend backward, and rotate. Static holding stretches improve the flexibility of the muscle in the direction stretched. ROM exercises remind muscles of their normal motions and stimulate correct muscle repair. ROM exercises also increase the production of fluids that lubricate the joints, which helps to maintain the strength and flexibility of the joints. ROM exercises can stimulate the repair of old muscle tears or strains even years after the injury.

COORDINATION OR AGILITY

A fourth major component of an exercise program is the development of neuromuscular coordination, also called "agility." Sports that require eye-hand coordination fine-tune the connection between nerve signals and muscle response. Balancing activities, such as walking across a beam or log, also spur nerve-muscle coordination. Gymnasts refine this exercise proficiency to an art form. Yoga routines usually include at least one balance exercise to develop this skill.

Early in our childhood development, we moved unilaterally. Our right hand moved forward with our right leg when we first learned to crawl.

Babies reach an important developmental milestone when they begin to "cross-crawl," moving the right arm with the left leg. Moving opposing limbs stimulates a variety of nerve centers in the brain. As adults, we still benefit from practicing cross-crawl movements.

MEDITATION IN MOTION

Exercise benefits the body in so many ways you could call it the "elixir of life." In addition to increasing fitness, exercise can be a profound meditation. Rhythmic movement combined with a meditative focus can transport you into other realms.

Walking is an excellent movement to begin practicing meditation in motion. Vipassana retreats routinely include walking meditation as part of the daily practice.

When you first practice walking meditation, move *slowly*. Become aware of your right heel striking the ground, the left toes pushing off. Note how the right quadricep muscles tighten as you shift weight onto the right foot. Feel the biceps muscles in the left leg complete the backward pulse. Become aware of the intricacy of the anatomy that moves you. Your movements will automatically slow as you deeply observe your body.

The point of walking meditation is to allow your physical movements to wholly consume your attention. Right here. Right now. Heel striking, toes pushing. Right now. Right here. Foot flat, other leg slowly drifting forward.

Sylvia Boorstein offers the following instructions for walking meditation in her book, *Don't Just Do Something, Sit There.* This form of moving meditation can be a wonderful ally, especially for those who have difficulty sitting for long periods of time.

Basic Instructions for Formal Walking Meditation

Pick a place to walk back and forth that is private and uncomplicated—one where the walking path can be ten to twenty feet long. If you walk outdoors, find a secluded spot so that you won't feel self-conscious. If you walk indoors, find a furniture-free section of your room or an empty hallway. Then you can devote all your attention to the feelings in your feet as you walk.

Keep in mind that this is attentiveness practice and tranquility practice, not specialty walking practice. You don't need to walk in any unusual way. No special balance is needed, no special graceful-ness. This is just plain walking. Perhaps at a slower pace than normal, but otherwise quite ordinary.

Begin your period of practice by standing still for a few moments at one end of your walking path. Close your eyes. Feel your whole body standing. Some people start by focusing their attention on the top of the head, then move their attention along the body through the head, shoulders, arms, torso, and legs, and end by feeling the sensations of the feet connecting with the earth. Allow your attention to rest on the sensations in the soles of the feet. This is likely to be the feeling of pressure on the feet and perhaps a sense of "soft" or "hard," depending on where you are standing.

Begin to walk forward. Keep your eyes open so that you stay balanced. I often begin with a normal strolling pace and expect that the limited scope of the walk, and its repetitious regularity, will naturally ease my body into a slower pace. Slowing down happens all by itself. I think it happens because the mind, with less stimuli to process, shifts into a lower gear. Probably the greed impulse, ever on the lookout for something novel to play with, surrenders when it realizes you're serious about not going anywhere.

When you walk at a strolling pace, the view is panoramic and descriptive. When your walking slows, the view is more localized and subjective. If we could see running readouts, like subtitles, of the mental notes that accompany walking, they might look like this:

Strolling pace: "Step . . . step . . . step . . . step . . . arms moving . . . head moving . . . smiling . . . looking . . . stopping . . . turning . . . bird chirping . . . stepping . . . stepping . . . wondering what time it is . . . thinking this is boring . . . stepping . . . stepping . . . swinging arms . . . feeling warm . . . feeling cool . . . I'm glad I'm in the shade . . . deciding to stay in the shade . . . smiling . . . stepping . . ."

Slower pace: "Pressure on feet . . . pressure . . . pressure disappearing . . . pressure reappearing . . . pressure shifting . . . lightness . . . heaviness . . . lightness . . . heaviness . . . lightness . . . Hey! Now I've got it! I'm finally present! . . . Whoops, I've been distracted . . . Start again . . . Pressure on the feet . . . pressure shifting . . .

lightness . . . heaviness . . . lightness . . . heaviness . . . hearing . . .
warm . . . cool . . ."

Slow is not better than fast. It's just different. Everything
changes, regardless of pace, and direct, firsthand experience of tem-
porality can happen while you are strolling just as much as while
you are stepping deliberately and slowly. The speed-limit guide for
mindful walking is to select the speed at which you are most likely to
maintain attention. Shift up or down as necessary.[10]

Mantra with Walking Meditation

You can also add a mantra or prayer that synchronizes with your movements. I recently backpacked out of the Haleakala Crater in Hawaii. After
three days of fasting and several miles of backpacking, I knew I would need
more than physical strength to carry me three thousand feet up the clifflike
edge of the crater.

I awoke the morning of the ascent to rain lashing against the tent. I
gathered and packed my sodden gear and hiked through driving rain and
wind to the base of the cliff. Water ran in rivulets over the rocks; the trail
was transformed into a streambed.

Thankfully the gusts of wind pushed me toward the cliff face. I began to
place my boots rhythmically—step, pause; step, pause—on the steep trail.

The rhythm began to carry me. I passed another hiker. Step, pause. Step,
pause. I was acutely aware of the elements—wind, water, rock. Only fire
was missing. Despite my rain gear, I was soaked to the skin and *cold.*

I remembered fire walking years before and how our guide had
instructed us to vibrate at the same frequency as the fire.

"Fire can't hurt you if you are one with the fire. If you vibrate at the
same rate, you are safe."

"OK," I told myself, "vibrate at the same frequency as wind and rain.
Become wind and rain. Then the elements can't hurt me. I am wind (foot
lands), I am water (foot lands). I am wind, I am water."

The chant continued to grow. "I am wind, I am water, I am rock. . .fire."

In truth, I *am* the elements. As long as I am in physical form, I am nothing more, nothing less than an arrangement of elements.

As I climbed, I sensed I was drawing elemental power through the soles
of the boots into the soles of my feet, into the soul of my being. For two

days after emerging from the crater, the chant continued to ring in my awareness. I've come to know its truth in the cells of my body.

I share this story to illustrate how you can create your own chant, inspired by a particular need or circumstance. You can also rely on traditional mantras or prayers to lift and carry you. The following list is not exhaustive, but rather a beginning point to ignite your interest and imagination:

- Hail, Mary, full of grace (Catholic)

- Quan Se An Bo Zi (Quan Yin, Goddess of Compassion, "She who hears the cries of the world.")

- Om Nama Shivaya

- Ischk Allah Mabud Leila (Sufi: All is the dance between the lover and the beloved.)

- Om Mane Pad Me Hum (Buddhist: The jewel in the lotus)

- Om Tare, Tu Tare, Ture Swaha (Tibetan Buddhism: Praise to Tara, Praise to Mother, I surrender.)

- The earth is our mother, we will take care of her. The earth is our mother, we will take care of her. Her sacred ground we walk upon, with every step we take. Her sacred ground we walk upon, with every step we take.

Besides walking, other examples of rhythmic exercise include swimming, biking, canoeing (on a lake or slow stretch of river), and inline skating. Experiment with your favorite forms of movement (doesn't "movement" sound less threatening than "exercise"?)

Swimming, for example, allows me to slip into a fluid motion. After several laps, I am just consciousness moving through water. The edges of my body are soft, my awareness diffuse. I am light slicing through water, making a ripple with my body, hardly disturbing the sea of life.

Seek a steady beat. Allow the repetition to carry you into a larger awareness and link you with celestial as well as earthly rhythms.

Reflections by Carol Lee Flinders

Carol Lee Flinders is an independent scholar and lecturer whose work as a writer began when she coauthored the classic Laurel's Kitchen *books on natural foods and vegetarianism. Today she writes primarily about women's spirituality—most recently in her new book* Enduring Lives: Portraits of Women and Faith in Action. *She lives in Northern California with her husband, Tim.*

I had of course been told about hot flashes and interrupted sleep, but nobody can really prepare you for how they feel! Both went on for several years. It's been blessedly over for maybe eight years now—I'm 62—and they were indeed vexing. But several things made it much easier to deal with them than they might have been, and they all have directly to do with my spiritual tradition.

My meditation teacher, Sri Eknath Easwaran, was of course a Hindu by upbringing, and he brought the wealth of that tradition to all his students— that is to say, a grounding in the Upanishads, the Bhagavad Gita, the great epics—lots of story in addition to direct teaching. And out of that we've absorbed so much: on the one hand, a deep insistence that we are not our bodies, that the body is my loyal and basically uncomplaining servant, and it's my job to take care of it well, and be grateful for everything it does for me; but, on the other hand, not to be driven by its needs or feel compulsively identified with it. It's not easy to acquire the full level of detachment that position would suggest, but even having come some of the way makes it so much easier to handle aging in general and the particular burden of losing one's dewy, delicious youthfulness in a culture that so idealizes the beauty of the young.

The Indian tradition teaches us that life has its stages, and that we should welcome each in its turn and live it out fully so that we don't look back full of regrets. But the tradition also teaches that we should always be preparing, all the time, for the stage that's coming up. That means that even as a young woman I live, ideally, in full recognition that my agility and complexion and figure and boundless energy may not always be there, but that other gifts will come along in their place. We're so impoverished here in contemporary Western society as far as that understanding is concerned.

I've loved being the age I am now. I couldn't have anticipated the burst of postmenopausal vitality and insight that came along right in the middle of the hot flashes. I've done my most satisfying work this last fifteen years—a string of four books that managed to say things that I'd have thought were buried too deep inside me to "get at." I'm so grateful for that. Oddly, it was with menopause that I was finally able to find my own voice.

You know, there is something so powerful about accepting that your womb is being decommissioned! I think it might be very tough if one weren't fully trusting that one's capacity to nurture and create—give birth even—hadn't moved to a different and ultimately more satisfying level. Teresa of Avila was very aware of that—she loved to use the language of enclosure and gestation to help her nuns realize that this was the work they were about, there in their cells, meditating.

More specifically, my teacher came from a matrilinear tradition, which means as he put it, "Not only were name and property handed down from grandmother to mother to daughter, but spiritual awareness itself flowed down the mother-line like a river." The imagery of flow itself seems to me deeply embedded in women's spirituality all over the world, and menstruation is right in the center of that network of symbols. Its cessation with menopause is really only about the body, though. The real flow has to do with grace, and lovingkindness—compassion that is meant to be boundless, beginning perhaps with our immediate relationships, but ultimately uncontainable.. . .

The discipline that helped me in particular, besides meditation itself, which is my rock, is the use of the "mantram," or holy name. It was through repetition of the mantram that I got through those sleepless nights and learned not to be afraid of them.

To learn more about Carol's writing and about her scheduled workshops, retreats, and lectures, visit her website at www.tworock.org.

CHAPTER ELEVEN

AN ADDITIVE APPROACH to BONE HEALTH: INNER and OUTER SUPPORT STRUCTURES

HUMANS, ALONG WITH ALL MAMMALS, CARRY OUR STRUCTURAL SUPPORT, our skeletal system, internally. Most insects have "exoskeletons," outer shells that protect the soft innards. In contrast, we mammals drape our muscles and other soft structures over and around the bones.

This elegantly designed support system also serves as the storage site for calcium and other important nutrients. Most of our exploration in this chapter focuses on maximizing bone density, the mineral packed into the bone. In truth, though, the bones are in a state of constant flux. Our bones release calcium and other nutrients into the bloodstream as needed. Simultaneously the blood delivers minerals to the bone for storage.

Our skeletal system supports our physical structure, while our moral and spiritual beliefs shape our inner environment. Like our bones, this internal structure is in a state of flux as we absorb the lessons gleaned from experience, and release that wisdom back into the world. At the end of this chapter, we will explore the "bones" that provide structure and support for our inner lives.

AN ADDITIVE PROGRAM FOR BUILDING HEALTHY BONES

Got a bone to pick?

Our bones are made of two major components: osteocalcin and minerals. Osteocalcin is a spongy, flexible connective-tissue matrix into which the minerals are embedded. Most of our discussion so far has focused on mineral content, but osteocalcin is equally important to bone health. Rather than being inert, rocklike substances, our bones actually flex and "give" slightly. This spongy, connective tissue matrix may explain why traditional women in South Africa have a low hip-fracture rate despite also having very low bone-mineral density.[1] Presumably healthy osteocalcin protects the bones against fracturing.

Although osteocalcin integrity is just as important as the amount of mineral packed into the bone, we have no way of measuring osteocalcin health. Current tests track only bone-mineral density. As the old saying goes, if you only have a hammer, everything looks like a nail. The current "hammer" for osteoporosis testing is the bone-mineral-density (BMD) scan, so almost all our research focuses on bone mineral content. Very little research addresses osteocalcin because we have no testing method for this important part of the bone. Keep in mind that while much of our discussion will center on BMD, the spongy connective tissue matrix is equally important.

As mentioned in chapter 8, we have two types of bone, trabecular and cortical. Trabecular bone is the inner part that includes the bone marrow. The "architecture," or structure, of trabecular bone prevents compression under pressure. Lack of physical exercise, low estrogen levels, and steroid use contribute to trabecular bone loss.

Cortical bone is a hard, circular, protective outer layer that protects the bone from trauma. This bone layer turns over at a much slower rate than trabecular bone, which is much more metabolically active. Low calcium and vitamin D levels most significantly impact the cortical bone.

The extremities (leg and arm bones) are 90 percent cortical bone. In contrast, the heel is made exclusively of trabecular bone. The hip bones are 50 percent trabecular and 50 percent cortical, while the spine is 90 percent trabecular and 10 percent cortical. Ideally a BMD scan tests hip and spine to accurately assess both trabecular and cortical bone health.

Bone and a Woman's Life Cycle

From the time we are born, we build more bone than we lose, finally reaching peak bone-mineral density between thirty-five and forty years old. After age forty, we begin to break down more bone than we rebuild, losing about 0.5 to 1.0 percent bone mass per year. For eight to ten years after menopause, bone loss increases by 2 to 5 percent per year.[1] The rate of loss slows again after age sixty-five.

For bone health, an ounce of prevention truly is more effective than a pound of cure. The best time to prevent osteoporosis is during the formative years, before age thirty-five. The higher our peak bone-mineral density in our mid- to late-thirties, the smaller our risk of bone fracture later in life.

The good news is that you can still prevent and sometimes even reverse bone loss even after menopause. How responsive your bones will be, and how aggressive you must be in order to impact bone health, depends on your particular body and your overall state of health. You can monitor your progress by repeating the BMD scan at regular intervals, for example, every one to three years.

The easiest ways to develop osteoporosis:

- Eat a Standard American Diet (SAD).

- Avoid exercise at all costs.

- Drink sweetened colas.

- Eat meat at every meal.

- Live in a polluted urban or industrial area.

- Smoke cigarettes.

- Drink lots of alcohol.

Making Choices that Support Bone Health

Rather than offering a one-size-fits-all program, this chapter outlines five progressive steps you can take to bolster bone health. If you are menopausal, have no family history of osteoporosis, and have already had a BMD scan that shows little or no bone-mineral loss, you may be able to maintain bone health and prevent osteoporosis simply by concentrating on steps 1 and 2 (nutrition and exercise). If, however, testing confirms mild to moderate bone loss, you may need to add steps 3 and 4. Women with severe bone loss would include all five steps in their bone restoration program.

This is an "additive" program, meaning each step provides the foundation for the next. You cannot effectively take supplements (step 3) and then ignore diet and exercise (steps 1 and 2). Similarly hormones (step 4) alone cannot support healthy bones. Start with the foundation and then add steps as needed to optimize bone health.

The Foundation: Nutrition and Exercise for Healthy Bones

These two lifestyle choices—nutrition and exercise—are both so crucial that I have placed them together to emphasize their equal importance in supporting bone health.

STEP 1: NUTRITION TO BUILD HEALTHY BONES

Most nutritional advice for bone health focuses on increasing calcium intake and absorption. The truth, though, is that calcium *loss* can have an even greater impact on bone health. We will also explore the myth that calcium builds strong bones. The truth is that calcium works in concert with many nutrients to build bone.

Acid-forming Foods that Encourage Bone Loss:

- Caffeine

- Sugar

- Alcohol

- High protein, especially animal protein

- High sodium

Besides sodium, all of these foods increase acidity. The body works very hard to maintain a steady pH level. As soon as pH in the bloodstream drops even slightly, the body immediately tries to buffer the increased acidity. The easiest, most readily available buffer is calcium, handily stored in large quantities in the bone. The more acidic our blood pH, the more calcium we leach from our bones to buffer that acidity.

Foods that Support Bone Health:

- Plant sources of protein (for example, whole grains and beans)

- Plant sources of calcium and other minerals

- Adequate protein intake during developing years

We absolutely need protein during childhood and early adult years to build healthy bones. Later in life, however, too much protein encourages bone loss. Animal protein sources have more sulfur-containing amino acids than plants, which means animal proteins have more of an acidifying effect in the body.

Plant sources of calcium and other minerals are easier to digest and absorb than animal sources. Although vegetables usually contain fewer minerals by volume, the body can absorb a higher percentage of those nutrients. As an example, we absorb 65 percent of the calcium in green cabbage but only 32 percent of the calcium in cow's milk.

How much protein should I be getting every day?

The World Health Organization recommends 40 to 50 grams of protein a day for adult men and women, or 0.6 g/kg of body weight. People who do hard physical labor require more protein, about 60 to 70 grams per day. Most Americans, however, particularly meat eaters, consume far more than 40 to 50 grams of protein a day. Some stray into the "pharmacological" range of 100 to 150 grams of protein a day, which is far beyond optimal range.

The Protein Myth and Bone Health: Is Protein Dissolving Your Bones?

Our digestive system breaks down protein into sulfur-containing compounds called uric acid or urea. The kidneys must metabolize and excrete these waste products; hence a high protein diet puts extra strain on the kidneys.

As mentioned earlier, uric acid also increases the acidity of the bloodstream, and the body pulls calcium from the bones to buffer the increased acidity. We have known since 1920 that a high protein diet, particularly a high animal-protein diet, causes more calcium to be excreted in the urine.[2] The amount of calcium dumped in the urine has the greatest impact on bone health. Calcium loss affects bone density more dramatically than calcium intake or calcium absorption.[3] In other words, the amount of calcium we *lose* impacts bone health more dramatically than the amount of calcium we *absorb*. A high protein diet that exceeds the normal physiological window taxes our bones as well as our kidneys.

Animal and plant proteins have different effects on the body. Animal proteins have more sulfur-containing amino acids, which increase acidity in the body. Methionine, a sulfur-containing amino acid particularly high in meats, eggs, and dairy products, is converted to homocysteine. Elevated homocysteine levels may increase bone loss. Plant proteins, in contrast, contain a very small percentage of these sulfur-containing amino acids and do not have the same acidifying effect in the body. The following chart compares a diet of animal protein only, a combination of animal and plant protein, and plant protein only.[4]

PROTEIN SOURCE	CALCIUM EXCRETION (MILLIGRAMS/DAY)
Beef, fish, chicken	150
Soy milk, eggs, textured vegetable protein	21
Soy milk, textured vegetable protein	103

A vegan diet (plant protein only) causes one-third less calcium loss than the animal protein diet. For women with moderate to severe osteoporosis, drastically reducing or eliminating animal proteins can help slow bone loss.

Colas Are "Bone Bombs"

Carbonated drinks contain a significant amount of phosphorus, which can compete with calcium and other minerals for absorption in the digestive tract. Sweetened colas also contain sugar and caffeine, both of which are implicated in reducing bone-mineral density.[5,6] Middle-aged women with long- term high caffeine intake have an increased risk for hip fracture. Among teen-aged girls, the more cola beverages consumed per week, the higher their rate of bone fracture later in life. In another study, the more soft drinks children consumed per week, the lower their serum calcium levels— in other words, they had less calcium in their blood to pack into their bones.[7] I call sweetened colas, those that combine phosphorus, sugar, and caffeine in one neat package, "bone bombs" because of their potentially devastating effect on our bones.

In Step 3 below, we will discuss specific nutrients and bone health.

STEP #2: EXERCISE TO BUILD HEALTHY BONES

Our bones must be "stressed" in order to catalyze bone building. The force of gravity and muscle movement are the most beneficial "stresses" on the bone. Each muscle contraction pulls against and slightly traumatizes the bone. This trauma signals the bone in that area to rebuild. During the rebuilding process, the bone packs new mineral into the osteocalcin, thereby increasing bone-mineral density and strengthening itself in the process.

Without movement, the bones never get the message to rebuild. You may absorb lots of minerals from your diet and/or supplements, but if you do not exercise, the bones never get the message to pack those minerals into the bone.

Exercise to Build and Maintain Strong Bones

Although women reach peak bone-mineral density between ages thirty-five and forty, the best time to prevent osteoporosis is in our teens and twenties. Exercise during these early years increases bone-mineral density and helps maximize our midlife peak. Women who continue a lifelong exercise program retain bone mass throughout their lives and have lower risk of fracture in later years.[8, 9] Increasing peak bone-mineral density by as little as 7 to 8 percent and then maintaining that increase through continued exercise reduces our risk of hip fracture up to five times.[10] Once we have reached peak bone-mineral density, we can help protect bone strength by continuing to exercise regularly.[11] For postmenopausal women, the largest increases in bone-mineral density are among women who are very physically active.[12] Yes, you read correctly. Even after menopause, women can potentially increase bone mass.

Moderate- versus High-Intensity Exercise

Low to moderate intensity exercise at best maintains bone-mineral density and may actually trigger bone loss rather than remineralization. Remember that physical stress signals bone cells to begin rebuilding. The bones seem to have a predetermined set point of damage or "deformation" (0.1 to 0.5 percent) that signals the bone to deposit more mineral than is removed. If deformation falls below the set point, the opposite occurs, that is, the bone loses more mineral than it deposits.[13, 14]

This set-point theory may explain why higher impact exercise, for example, running and weight lifting[15, 16], stimulates greater increases in bone-mineral density than more moderate forms of exercise such as walking or swimming.(17)

Weight-Bearing Exercise

Weight-bearing exercise refers to movement that places pressure on the bone, either from the weight of the body or the force of a muscle contraction. "Weight bearing" does not necessarily mean "weight lifting," although weight lifting is one example of weight-bearing exercise. Any activity that places weight on the femur (thigh bone), hips, and spine qualifies as weight-bearing exercise. Other examples include walking, jogging, running, gymnastics, and some sports (for example, basketball and volleyball).

Most general recommendations for bone health focus on weight-bearing exercise to increase bone-mineral density. Remember that exercise intensity is as important as the type. Both jogging and walking, for example, are forms of weight-bearing exercise. Jogging exerts more pressure on the bone and therefore is a higher intensity form of weight-bearing exercise than walking.

For many older women, however, high-impact weight-bearing exercise can damage joints and/or increase the risk of fracturing already fragile bones. The good news is that some studies suggest that moderate weight-bearing exercise, such as riding a stationary bike[18] and swimming[19], increase bone density as well, although not to as great a degree as some of the higher intensity forms of exercise.

Strength-Building Exercise and Strong Bones

Strong muscles support strong bones. The stronger the muscle, the more forceful the contraction or "pull" against the bone. According to the set-point model, a stronger muscle contraction would be more likely to reach the threshold to stimulate bone remineralization.

Some women in weight-lifting programs increase bone-mineral density only in the areas exercised,[20] while others have a more generalized increase.[21] As an example of a localized effect, increased physical activity improves back-muscle strength and enhances bone-mineral density in the lumbar (lower) spine.[22]

Perhaps you have not exercised regularly for many years and have never lifted weights. Are you wondering if starting to exercise now would make a difference? Thankfully the answer is a whole-hearted "Yes!" Even elderly nursing home residents (ages eighty-six to ninety-six) significantly benefited from a weight-training program using low weights and many repetitions.[23] Gradual weight training can increase both muscle mass and bone-mineral density.

A Balanced Exercise Program

A good exercise program includes all four types of exercise (endurance, flexibility, strength building, and coordination) either within one exercise session or over the course of a week.

Endurance: Remember the FIT (Frequency, Intensity, Time) concept. For minimum cardiovascular fitness, exercise aerobically three times a week for twenty minutes at your target heart rate.

Stretch: For at least five minutes a day.

Strength Building: Include strength-building exercise three times a week.

Agility: At least two minutes of coordination or balancing exercise each day, which could be flipping a Frisbee with the kids or doing a balancing yoga posture such as The Tree.

TOTAL TIME PER WEEK (to maintain basic fitness): 170 minutes. That translates to an average of 25 minutes a day, probably less time than you spend watching your favorite news program or sit-com! To increase bone-mineral density, you will need to increase the intensity and duration of your exercise program.

Tips for Starting an Exercise Program

Choose types of exercise you love.

The activities you most enjoy can be wonderful sources of exercise. "You mean dancing counts as exercise?" asked one incredulous patient. "Of course," I told her, "as long as you are moving steadily, increasing your heart rate, and breathing deeply. You can even dance in your own living room."

Incorporate exercise into your daily life.

The easier your routine, the more likely you will be to continue exercising. You don't necessarily have to squeeze into Lycra tights and drive across town to a gym to exercise. Of course if you enjoy exercise clubs, by all means join a club. If you live far away from an exercise gym or don't like the atmosphere, you can discover many other ways to include exercise in your daily routine. If you live in town, consider walking to the post office or grocery store instead of driving. Walk the dog twice a day instead of once; perhaps over time the pace can increase to a jog or a run. Work in the garden. Rake leaves. Shovel snow, one of the most challenging, strength-building, aerobic exercises around! Play your favorite music and dance in the living room, with or without your sweetie. Check out exercise videos at the public library.

Begin slowly!

Many enthusiastic people beginning a new exercise program push themselves too hard the first day or week. The first day the body often seems remarkably fit. You may easily surpass your initial goals. Twenty-four to forty-eight hours after that first walk or weight-lifting session, however, you may vow never to don your sweats again. At that point, sore muscles and aching joints may be painful reminders of your overexertion.

I really do mean "slowly."

Someone who has not exercised for years, for example, might begin with a five-minute walk every day. The second week increase to a seven-minute walk, the third week to eight or nine minutes a day. Better to begin with small, attainable goals and gradually increase activity than experience the agony of running three miles the first day out. Suddenly exerting the body increases the likelihood of damaging a joint, tearing a muscle, or overtaxing the heart.

If you cannot find a continuous block of time to exercise, break up your exercise program into smaller time segments. An example for the Wonder Woman Working Mom:

♦ Walk the dog for five minutes in the morning, followed by five minutes of yoga stretches (for example, Salute to the Sun). If you don't have a dog, take a short walk anyhow (or borrow the neighbor's dog).

♦ Park as far away from the office building as possible and walk across the parking lot.

♦ Use stairs instead of the elevator.

♦ Spend five minutes climbing stairs during lunch, or take a five-minute walk.

♦ In the afternoon, instead of a five-minute coffee break, climb the stairs again.

♦ In the evening, lift light dumb-bells while watching TV

For those able to exercise for an extended period, warm up for at least five minutes at the beginning of an exercise session.

Stretch gently, or simply begin whatever exercise you are doing at a slower pace. Begin walking slowly for five minutes, for example, then step up the pace to reach your target heart rate. Warming the muscles reduces later muscle soreness and decreases the likelihood of muscle tears.

Slow your pace at the end of each exercise session.
This slow-down period allows your heartbeat and breathing to return to normal. Stopping exercise suddenly may cause blood to pool in the legs and lead to fainting. Continue moving, just reduce your speed.

If you are sore, gentle exercise relieves muscle pain more
effectively than analgesics (for example, aspirin).
Take a short walk and do a series of gentle stretching exercises. Immediate muscle soreness probably is caused by increased acidity (lactic acid) and prostaglandin production. Delayed onset muscle soreness (twenty-four to

forty-eight hours after exercising) probably is caused by micro-tears in the muscle and connective tissue. Stretching reminds the muscle tissue of its normal function so that the muscle fibers repair in the right direction. Muscles repaired without gentle stretching are more likely to form a mass of criss-crossing fibers, or "scar" tissue, that does not function normally.

Always do less than you think you can, particularly
in the first month of an exercise program.
Give your body time to adjust to new activities. Remember you are making changes for a lifetime. If you need an extra month to reach your weight-lifting target, who's counting? You will be enjoying the benefits of your exercise program for decades to come, not just in the coming weeks and months.

Vary the type of exercise.
Choose at least three different types of exercise you enjoy and rotate among them at regular intervals. Aerobic training is specific to the muscle groups exercised. In other words, running five miles a day develops aerobic fitness, but if you switch to bicycle riding, you will not have as great an aerobic capacity on the bike as you did running. Your body increases aerobic capacity in conjunction with the specific muscles you are training. This research spawned "cross-training" programs to develop multiple muscle groups and enhance aerobic training/capacity.

Boning Up for a Lifetime of Health
Exercise is a powerful ally in building and maintaining bone health. No matter what your age, moderate- to high-intensity exercise will benefit your bones. If you are pursuing your vision of health, the changes you make now are more likely to last for a lifetime.

Step 3: Supplements to Build Bone
Although calcium has enjoyed the most attention, all of the following nutrients are vital for bone health.

CALCIUM FOOD SOURCES
Have the billboards with milk-moustached movie stars swayed you to drink more milk? Although high in calcium, milk may not be your best ally in building bone.

Genetic researchers consider northern Europeans' ability to digest milk throughout their life cycle a genetic aberration or adaptation rather than the norm. On a global scale, most of us can digest milk only until age two or three, and human milk is the milk of choice. Each animal's milk stimulates different types of growth. Human milk, for instance, is high in essential fatty acids and stimulates brain and neural development. In contrast, a baby calf's first priority is to stand and walk, so cow's milk stimulates muscle development.

Estimated Percentage of Lactose Intolerance in Different Populations[24]

- Vietnamese 100%
- American Indian 95%
- Southern Italian 72%
- African American 65%
- Northern Italian 50%
- French 32%
- White Americans 22%
- Austrian 20%
- Northern European 7%
- Dutch 0%

Animal sources of calcium are also much more difficult for your body to assimilate than plant sources, as you can see from the following chart. Although lower in calcium, plant sources are easier for your body to absorb. One cup of Chinese cabbage, for example, delivers almost as much absorbable calcium as a cup of milk.

CALCIUM SUPPLEMENTS

If you are concerned about bone health, your physician may advise you to take an antacid that contains calcium carbonate (such as Tums). Unfortunately antacids are poor sources of calcium for two reasons:

- Calcium and all minerals need an acidic environment in the stomach to break down. Antacids by their very nature reduce stomach acidity. Elderly people often have more difficulty absorbing minerals and other nutrients because they produce less stomach acid.

CALCIUM ABSORPTION FROM SELECTED PLANT FOODS[25]

FOOD SOURCE	CALCIUM CONTENT	PERCENTAGE ABSORPTION	CALCIUM ABSORPTION
Beans, pinto (1/2 cup)	45	17	7.6
Broccoli (1/2 cup)	35	53	18.4
Brussels sprouts (1/2 cup)	19	64	12
Cabbage, Chinese (1/2 cup)	79	54	43
Cabbage, Green (1/2 cup)	25	65	16
Kale (1/2 cup)	47	59	28
Mustard greens (1/2 cup)	47	59	37
Sesame seeds (1 ounce)	28	21	7.7
Tofu, raw, firm (1/2 cup)	258	31	80
Turnip greens (1/2 cup)	99	52	51
Cow's milk (1 cup)	300	32	96

About 40 percent of postmenopausal women are severely deficient in stomach acid.[26] You can maximize absorption by taking mineral supplements with an acidic fruit juice (for example, grapefruit juice) or food.

♦ Calcium carbonate, made from seashells, is difficult for the digestive tract to break down and absorb. "Chelated" forms of minerals, that is, a mineral attached to an amino acid, are easier for the stomach to break down than minerals bound to other minerals. Examples of calcium chelates include calcium citrate, calcium malate, and calcium aspartate.

♦ See "How to Maximize Supplement Absorption" (p. XXX) for more information about how to maximize the benefit of all your supplements.

HOW MUCH CALCIUM DO I NEED?

Many menopausal women concerned about bone health ask me, "How much calcium should I take?"

"What other nutrients are you taking?" is my reply. "Calcium alone cannot build strong bones." When a patient looks mystified, I offer the following analogy: Imagine going to hear Beethoven's Ninth Symphony. When the curtain goes up, only one clarinetist is sitting on the stage. Of course one musician cannot play an entire symphony, just as one single nutrient cannot build strong bones.

Bone health depends on calcium, magnesium, all of the other minerals, and several vitamins as well. Supplementing a large quantity of a single nutrient may actually inhibit the absorption or function of another nutrient. Taking large amounts of calcium, for example, drives down magnesium supplies in the body. Calcium and magnesium compete for absorption in the intestines. Normally foods containing calcium also contain magnesium, so the body absorbs some of each nutrient.

The amount of calcium you need depends on your diet and the amount and variety of other nutrients you are supplementing. Recent research suggests taking too much calcium by itself can actually increase risk of hip fracture.[27, 28] Remember that in order for calcium to be absorbed and properly used in the body, *all* of the other nutrients must be present.

Postmenopausal women need approximately 1000 mg of calcium a day. If you are supplementing calcium citrate or malate, you can reduce that amount by one-quarter to one-half because these calcium supplements are more easily absorbed.

WHAT ABOUT THE RATIO OF CALCIUM TO MAGNESIUM?

We do not have a definitive answer about the best ratio of calcium to magnesium. Some studies suggest twice as much calcium as magnesium, others advocate equal amounts, and still others recommend twice as much magnesium as calcium. I recommend you supplement at least half as much magnesium as calcium. If you are taking 600 mg of calcium citrate, for example, you should take at least 300 mg of magnesium.

VITAMIN D

This vital bone-building nutrient increases calcium absorption in the intestines and deposition in the bones. When exposed to sunlight, cholesterol in our skin converts to vitamin D. Even twenty minutes of sun exposure in northern climates should be enough to generate sufficient quantities of vitamin D. Fish, eggs, and liver also contain significant amounts. Vegetarians who get little sun exposure may need to supplement vitamin D. Recommended amounts: 200 to 400 IU daily.

VITAMIN C
In addition to numerous other functions, vitamin C promotes the normal formation and cross-linking of proteins that make up part of our bones' structure. Recommended amounts: at least 1000 mg per day, divided into two or three doses.

MANGANESE
Manganese encourages the production of proteinlike molecules called "mucopolysaccharides." These saccharides form a base for calcium deposits in the bones. Without manganese, the body cannot pack calcium into the bones. Recommended amounts: 15 to 30 mg per day.

BORON
Boron is an important cofactor for the synthesis of testosterone and 17 beta-estradiol. In addition, supplementing boron reduces urinary loss of calcium and magnesium by 44 percent.[29] Recommended amounts: 3 mg per day.

B6, B12, AND FOLIC ACID
As mentioned above, high animal-protein intake can result in the formation of more homocysteine, an amino acid that has been linked with increased risk for osteoporosis and heart disease. Homocysteine normally converts to other less harmful byproducts if the body has adequate amounts of three important nutrients: B6, B12, and folic acid. Recommended amounts: 50 to100 mg of B6, 400 to 800 mcg folic acid, and 3 to15 mcg of B12.

ZINC
Important for many functions in the body, zinc enhances the activity of vitamin D. Zinc promotes the normal synthesis of DNA and protein, making it a vital nutrient for the formation of proteins in the bone, osteoblasts (bone builders), and osteoclasts (bone destroyers). Recommended amounts: 15 to 30 mg per day.

HOW TO MAXIMIZE SUPPLEMENT ABSORPTION

◆ Choose encapsulated or gel-cap supplements. Tablets can be very difficult for the stomach to break down, particularly mineral tablets. Digesting a hard-packed mineral tablet is a bit like trying to break down a pebble. The tablet may pass through the digestive tract unchanged.

◆ To determine whether your mineral tablet will break down: drop one mineral tablet in six ounces of room-temperature vinegar, and stir every two to three minutes. After thirty minutes the mineral tablet should have disintegrated into small particles. If the tablet has not broken down, do not use that supplement.

◆ Choose a good multivitamin and mineral supplement rather than a handful of single nutrients. The nutrients function best together, not in isolation.

◆ The Recommended Daily Allowance (RDA) aims to prevent major diseases, not promote optimal health. Each body has different nutritional requirements. Ask a health-care provider trained in nutrition what amounts of nutrients are optimal for you.

◆ Choose a multivitamin and mineral that requires four to six capsules per day. No one can squeeze an adequate amount of nutrients into a single multivitamin and mineral tablet or capsule.

◆ Avoid supplements that contain dyes and preservatives.

◆ If you have food allergies, read labels carefully. Many supplement manufacturers now list common food allergens such as corn, dairy, yeast, and wheat.

Step 4: Hormonal Bone Support

For women with moderate to severe bone loss, hormone replacement therapy (HRT) may effectively halt or reverse bone loss.

◆ Estrogen maintains bone that has already been build by blocking the activity of osteoclasts, cells that break down bone mineral. Estrogen has the most effect on trabecular bone.

♦ Progesterone stimulates osteoblasts, cells that lay down new bone mineral.

♦ Testosterone also stimulates osteoblasts. Although both progesterone and testosterone have the potential to increase bone-mineral density, I prefer to supplement progesterone because a woman's body is accustomed to higher progesterone than testosterone levels. If a woman has had her ovaries removed, however, her testosterone has dropped by 50 percent. In her case, I would most likely prescribe testosterone in addition to estrogen and progesterone.

Step 5: Pharmaceutical Drugs for Emergency Bone Care

The most commonly prescribed nonhormonal drug for osteoporosis is alendronate. Known by the trade name Fosamax, this and other bisphosphonates block the action of osteoclasts, cells that break down bone. When first introduced, bisphosphonates were meant to be used only for short-term treatment (six months or less). Phosphorus, an extremely volatile element, can chemically burn the digestive tract. Prescription inserts warn patients to remain upright for at least thirty minutes after swallowing a dose of the medication to prevent irritating the esophagus. With long-term use, Fosamax can cause a host of gastrointestinal symptoms including diarrhea, heartburn, and other GI tract irritation. In their favor, bisphosphonates do provide an alternative for women with moderate to severe bone loss who cannot take hormones.

Choosing Which Steps to Follow

Remember that your personal and family medical history offer important clues about your risk for developing osteoporosis. A bone-mineral density (BMD) scan can help assess the amount of mineral packed in the bone. The BMD scan can be repeated to track your progress and evaluate whether your treatment plan is aggressive enough to maintain or improve bone health.

Summary of Steps to Support Bone Health

1. Little or no bone loss: Diet and exercise (Steps 1 and 2).

2. Low to moderate loss: In addition to diet and exercise, add supplements (step 3) and possibly progesterone (step 4).

3. Moderate to high loss: In addition to diet, exercise, and supplements, add progesterone, estrogen, and possibly testosterone (step 4).

4. Severe loss: In addition to steps 1, 2, 3, and 4, consider short-term use of bisphosphonates (step 5).

MORAL STRUCTURE: THE BONES OF OUR INNER LANDSCAPE

In chapter 6, we explored the inner territories we traverse during transitional periods in our lives. We will take the opportunity now to explore the inner structures that support those landscapes.

According to Robert Fritz, a master of both personal and organizational structures, form follows structure. The river always flows along the path of least resistance. In other words, the internal structures we adopt guide the flow of our thoughts, our beliefs, and our behaviors.

In 1977, Rosabeth Moss Kanter won the C. Wright Mills award for *Men and Women of the Corporation,* her in-depth study of women's entry into the corporate world. In the early 1970s, many people assumed that corporate America would become a softer, more responsive place to work as more women entered the corporate workforce. In contrast, instead of creating "kinder, gentler" worksites, women adopted the same behaviors and attitudes as the men in the corporation. The corporate structure shaped the women's attitudes, beliefs, and behaviors.

The structures we inhabit in turn shape our internal landscapes. For the hijackers who destroyed the World Trade Center towers, for example, their actions were the natural outgrowth of their internal structures. Their actions were not so much a symptom of Islam as a religion, but rather the outcome of fundamentalist thinking. Fundamentalists of any stripe believe that everyone should conform to their particular way of thinking and behaving. This is the disease of "overcalcification" Just as ingesting too much calcium, without the balance of other nutrients, eventually leads to calcium deposition in unwanted areas, such as in muscle tissue and joint capsules, absorbing too much of a single idea or belief system can create rigid boundaries between self and others. The ideas "calcify" into walls that divide, instead of bridges that unite.

I am by no means encouraging people to abandon the spiritual beliefs that sustain their lives. Instead I am encouraging you to examine whether your beliefs unite you with spirit and other human beings, or whether they isolate you from others. Does your spirituality open your heart to Creator, humans, and the larger community of life? Does your spirituality encourage you to shun those with different belief systems or to associate with them only in hopes of converting them to your way of thinking? Are your beliefs rooted deeply enough that you can comfortably entertain another's beliefs without threatening your own?

Years ago I read accounts of the first missionaries who came to the New World to convert the "heathen" natives. Most of the native people who met the missionaries listened politely to the missionaries' descriptions of Jesus and their Christian God. They were trained to listen respectfully to visitors; they treated all guests with deference and respect, even those with differing ideas and beliefs.

After listening to the missionary, the native people tried to share their own view of spirituality, with the attitude "I've listened respectfully to you; now I will share my views with you." How shocked the native people must have been when their guest rudely interrupted and told them their beliefs were wrong.

Who am I to judge the details of another's relationship with Creator, as long as that union breeds respect and love for all of life?

I am not suggesting that everyone adopt a hodge-podge of spiritual beliefs and thereby develop one, homogenous world religion. Instead I am suggesting we adopt appreciation for other spiritual traditions while continuing to practice our own.

I had a housemate years ago who had discovered a way to end racism. "There should be a law that everyone has to marry someone of a different race," he explained triumphantly. "Eventually we would all look the same, and no one could point to another person and say, 'Hey, their skin color is different!'"

I appreciate the spirit of his insight; he wanted to eliminate the differences that, at least perceptually, divide us. From another turn of the spiral, however, we could eliminate the divisive *perception* and transform it into appreciation. "Yes, you are different, and I celebrate that difference." Instead of obliterating our physical and spiritual differences, we could revel in the rich tapestry of our diversity.

Setting Sail: Beliefs Guide Our Inner Passage

Age guarantees that eventually I will meet physical, mental, emotional, and spiritual challenges. When feeling strong and centered, I recognize those challenges as opportunities to strengthen my inner "muscles." When I am off balance, I can try to "duck" from those challenges, escaping from myself with alcohol or drugs, numbing myself with food, or shielding myself with self-righteous anger. In reality, though, I can never completely avoid those difficult emotions. They are temporarily swept under the carpet until I have the strength or wisdom to address them.

The internal structures I develop will determine how well I handle the inevitable difficulties I will encounter. I cannot control the outer circumstance; I can only influence my response to those conditions. Do my beliefs keep me supple and strong, agile and coordinated in my responses? Does my spirituality support self-pity, blame, or fear? Within my spiritual structure, am I a responsive participant or a victim of circumstances? Do the "bones" of my landscape provide support, or do they cripple my attempts to respond?

The Winds of Fate

One ship drives east, and another drives west
With the selfsame winds that blow.
'Tis the set of the sails
and not the gales
Which tells us the way to go.

Like the winds of the sea are the winds of fate
As we voyage along through life,
'Tis the set of the soul
That decides its goal
And not the calm or the strife.

—Ella Wheeler Wilcox[30]

Explore the "Bones" of Your Inner Structure

I grew up in a family that assumed being a Methodist and voting Republican was genetically determined. That double-helix spiraling in each cell, according to my relatives, governed my inner structure just as surely as my physical features.

How unsettling for my family that I received mutant genes; my spiritual biology did not match their own. I felt like the ugly duckling deposited in the swan's nest, the "mistaken zygote" so eloquently described in Clarissa Pinkola Estes' work.

Over many years I have gradually discerned commonalities in the core moral and spiritual beliefs we hold. Like my parents, I am deeply devoted to spirit. The outer expression differs: they are devoted to religion and God; I am devoted to Creator and spirituality. We are devoted to service and caring for others. We value scholarship and the cultivation of the mind, although the topics and methods vary. Reverence for the earth and all aspects of creation is a strong river running through my ancestry.

I offer you the following questions to explore your own beliefs, the structural supports for your own spirituality. This is an opportunity to review your familial inheritance (if any) and observe your own evolution.

- What spiritual or religious training did you receive as a child? Did you learn by example, from your parents or other family members? Did a neighbor take you to church or synagogue? Did you have formal religious training or participate in community ceremonies? Did your family have their own rituals and celebrations at home? In difficult situations, how did you cope? Did you learn to talk to God/Goddess/Creator/All That Is?

- What did you learn about other spiritual traditions? Were you encouraged to visit or learn about other religious groups? I remember asking my mother when I was seven years old to take me to visit other churches. Even at that age, I instinctively knew that I was searching for something more or perhaps something different from what I was receiving in my Sunday school education. "Why don't you spend more time at *our* church?" was my mother's reply.

- How did your beliefs deepen as you grew older? As your moral "bones" developed, what did you carry with you from childhood? How did that structure serve you as you matured?

- Did you continue within the same religious or spiritual tradition? Did you explore? What were the results of your exploration within your own tradition or within another? How did your relationship with spirit evolve?

♦ Have you found a community of like-hearted people to share your faith? Do you have spiritual mentors who can support you in continuing to deepen your path? Are you alone and isolated in your beliefs? How accepting is your larger community of differing spiritual and religious traditions?

♦ What do you value? What would you die for? Even more importantly, what would you *live* for, with all your heart and soul? What ignites your passion? What lights your world?

♦ What values are you modeling for your children, your grandchildren, your community? What morals and beliefs do you want to seed for the coming generations? How are you "planting" those beliefs, passing them on to others?

Years ago I visited Mesa Verde in southwestern Colorado and signed up for a tour of one of the cliff dwellings. A National Park Service ranger guided our group down the steep trail and into a cliff overhang that housed a carefully structured, ancient community. After showing us through the homes, food storage caches, and ceremonial kivas, he guided us into a tight circle. "Look at your hands," he instructed us. Each of us gazed into the fissured surfaces of our palms. "Everything you see here was created by hands," he said, carefully extending his palms toward us. "The ancient people used their hands to create this place." He spoke slowly, looking intently into each of our eyes. "With our hands, we can create or destroy. With our hands, we can hurt each other, or care for each other. The choice is yours." The simple depth and intensity of his message caught me by surprise. I wasn't expecting a moral lesson at the end of our tour. Tears sprang into my eyes. When we returned to the parking lot, I took a few moments to thank our guide and to express my appreciation for the message he was delivering to visitors in the park. He explained that during his thirty years of teaching in the public school system, he and other teachers had come together to create a program to teach morals and values. "Those lessons will stay with them long after they've forgotten geometry and physics," he explained. "Some kids weren't learning morals and values at home, so we developed a way of teaching them after school." After retirement, he looked for a way to combine his love of nature with his desire to teach morals and values. His summer job as a National Park ranger married those two passions. He had found an effective way of nurturing values in the current and future generations.

As you follow the river, continuing the journey through menopause into the next stage of your life, consider the structure that carries you. How healthy are your physical bones? What are you doing to nurture your physical foundation? Remember, too, to nurture your inner structures. Tend the beliefs, values, and morals that support your spiritual life. Adopt values and morals that engender a healthy spiritual posture, standing in alignment with the good of you and all of life.

Reflections by Dr. Beth Davis

Beth Davis, M.A., N.D., is a naturopathic doctor with a family practice in the small community of Madras, Oregon. Educator and doctor, she delights in encouraging health and healing on the mental, emotional, spiritual, and physical levels. She guides experiential workshops with her partner, Ruth Traut, in Earth Healing, Women's Mysteries and Rites of Passage, and Vision Quest. She and Ruth are currently establishing a healing and retreat center in central Oregon.

I really had no idea what menopause would be like. None of my female relatives shared their experience. It was, like so many things about being a woman, sort of a hush-hush subject. The only personal experience I had of someone going through menopause was in being around my mother as she went through it. She did not say what was happening. I did not put together what was happening until later when I thought of her age and her behavior. She was extremely volatile emotionally, one minute crying and the next angry. I never knew what mood she would be in when I returned home from school, which made me quite anxious. She seemed overly tired and somewhat depressed. She would often be napping when I came in from school and she would sleep until it was time to get up and make dinner for the family. Her course through menopause ended with a hysterectomy. When I, age eighteen, asked why she had needed the surgery, one of my aunts told me she had been bleeding very profusely for too long and the surgery would stop the bleeding.

Though I was not prepared for menopause, I looked forward to getting older. I felt that with age came certain freedoms. Freedom from having to look and act a certain way in order to be attractive to men or to be a proper lady. Growing up in Virginia, I may have gotten a different education on feminine behavior than girls in other parts of the country. Certainly, when I came out West as an adult, I felt women in the western states had much more freedom to be themselves than I had felt in the South.

The first sign of menopause that I noticed in myself was in the way my mind worked. All my life I had been good in school, so that my left brain was well developed. I could easily remember things, my memorization skills were good, I thought things through in a logical manner from point A to B to C and so forth. I have wanted to be a doctor since childhood, so I needed to get good grades in school and prove myself worthy intellectually. When menopause came along, I began to be unable to recall things, including people's names, a certain word I wanted to use, a description of a movie I had seen. I began to fear that I was losing my mental faculties that I had relied on throughout my life.

Worse, I had decided at age fifty to finally study medicine, and I wondered if I would be able to do the coursework with all the memorization. I decided to try, as it had been my dream to be a doctor for so many years. I did not want to let the opportunity pass me by. Now I believe those years of study strengthened my mind and that what was happening to my way of thinking was that the corpus collosum, which connects the two hemispheres of the brain, was growing and making a better connection between the left and right sides of the brain. I was learning how to use the right brain, the sphere of patterns, intuition, seeing the whole picture, music, and art. I believe this way of learning, seeing the whole, actually helped me in medical school because I could grasp concepts and see how they fit into the whole picture much more easily and quickly than I had before. My left-brain function was strong enough to see me through when rote memorization was called for and actually was aided by a more whole understanding of what I was learning because of the right-brain way of perceiving.

The other major change I experienced with my menopause was that I began to regain the sense of independence and self-confidence I had had as a prepubescent girl. I remember myself before puberty as doing what I wanted, following my own wishes, talking, dressing, acting like *me* without the awful sense that came with puberty that I was supposed to be a certain way because I was female. As a menopausal woman, I was released of those bonds and could be myself again.

I had few of the "usual" symptoms of menopause. Once in a while, I experienced a flush of heat for no reason, but I was spared the awful sweats and beet-red face and chest. Some joint pain did come up for me at this time, which is a genetic susceptibility for me. I also gained weight and found it harder to lose than before menopause. I have since learned that all of these symptoms are ones many women experience. I did not, thankfully, repeat my mother's mood swings, fatigue, or heavy bleeding. My periods just became irregular, shorter, and finally stopped when I was fifty-one years of age.

RITES OF PASSAGE FOR WOMEN

One of the best gifts of menopause for me was sitting in a circle of menopausal women and sharing experiences. Ruth Traut and I were leading a workshop in Germany entitled "Rites of Passage for Women." As part of the workshop, we had women break into small circles of those who were going through a certain passage of a woman's life. These passages we usually name following the old Celtic names of Maiden for first blood or menstruation, Mother for fertile woman giving birth to children or to a life work, Changing Woman for the menopause time, and Crone for the time of elderhood. I sat in a circle of nine menopausal women and for the first time in my life heard from other women about their menopause. With laughter and tears, we told our stories to each other. What a gift to have one's story witnessed! I found I was not the only one to feel that I was going back to the strength and independence of the young girl before menarche. We heard our commonalties and our differences, and grew in respect for ourselves as women. It was pure joy to be with these women.

When Ruth and I offer these workshops on "Rites of Passage" or "Women's Mysteries," we never do the same thing twice. The workshops are experiential and are built upon the individual women who are there and their particular stories. We usually talk at the beginning about the many changes women go through in their lives—from young girl, to menstruation, to fertility and motherhood, to the cessation of bleeding, to old age and death. Those passages have not been honored in our lifetimes as they have been in earlier ages on the earth (four to five thousand years ago). We talk of those times in human history when the feminine was honored for its qualities of fertility, nurturance, intuition, emotion, spirituality, receptivity; how qualities of woman were equated with qualities of the moon and the earth. The feminine has not been honored in our lifetimes and that has not only hurt us as women, but it has also hurt the male of the species and the earth. We talk about the need to bring back the feminine energy to the human and planetary community. We talk about our need as individual women to honor ourselves and thus our mothers and daughters and all women; that it is very much our duty and pleasure to rebirth respect for the feminine in the present time.

From that beginning, we facilitate talking circles, experiences with the earth and the moon, dances, chants, and small circles for sharing their experiences as women and thus seeing their lives more clearly. From these sharings, small groups create a ceremony to celebrate their particular rite of passage or time of life. These ceremonies are offered to the whole circle at the end of the workshop. We find that sharing the pain and shame, the joy, the fear, the disappointments, forgiveness and acceptance, and the sense of community that grows among us, are all important to the potency of the ceremonies the women create. And what wondrous ceremonies they are!

At each of the "Rites of Passage for Women," we have been blessed to have women from age twelve to late seventies. It is such a pleasure to see how young and old listen and learn from each others' stories. It is something I missed as a girl and young woman. It feels very good to have a small part in bringing that gift to girls and women today. It is a very personal gift for me each and every time.

Beth can be contacted at: 227 S.E. 6th Street, PO Box 513, Madras, OR 97741; Phone: (541) 475-5525; Fax: (541) 475-5525; Email: drbethnd@madras.net

CHAPTER TWELVE

RITUAL to MARK the MENOPAUSAL JOURNEY: RITES and CELEBRATIONS

CONTEMPORARY WESTERN CULTURE HAS FEW RITUALS TO MARK RITES OF passage. Without a living tradition to guide us in making life changes, some of us unconsciously create our own. Teenagers who do not have ceremonies to mark their passage into adult years, for example, create their own "celebrations," sometimes in very unhealthy ways: drugs, drinking, sex, and fast cars. In traditional "primary" cultures, a youth might be tested physically and spiritually. A young Navaho woman would mark her first moontime bleeding by running long distances for several days. Young Lakota men (and sometimes women) would complete a vision quest, fasting and praying for vision. These rites of passage develop both physical and spiritual endurance. The ceremony itself requires the young person to *create* new inner resources. They may also discover reserves and talents previously unrecognized in themselves.

These ceremonies prepare the individual as well as the community for a new phase of life. Traditional puberty ceremonies offer an opportunity for children to transform into adults—both in their own eyes and in the perception of the larger community.

And what ceremonies do women have to mark the transition from adult to elder, from reproductive to inwardly productive years? I know of very few cultures that mark and honor this transition. Like the undirected youth, many of us turn to less-than-healthy ways of addressing the aging process. We have affairs, join rock bands, buy convertible sports cars, take up marathon running, have a face lift, tuck our tummies, or move to Venezuela.

All of the frenetic outward activity shields us from inner changes our soul may want to make. After so many years of outwardly directed activity, building a career and/or raising children, that inward focus may feel awkward, like the gawky arrangement of long legs, newly sprouted breasts, and pubic hair that signal our youth. This time, though, the transformation rests more in our souls than in our physicality.

This awkwardness is like the plump caterpillar hanging upside down, surrendering to some unfathomable inner prompting, and beginning to spin the chrysalis for its new life from its own flesh and blood. At some point during its sojourn in the cocoon, that caterpillar completely liquefies before reconstituting itself as "butterfly."

How many of us are prepared for such a journey, completely abandoning our familiar forms, and surrendering to a completely new way of being and living? If we are courageous enough to adopt the caterpillar's faith, the menopausal journey can offer such an experience. Certainly menopause is not the only opportunity for profound transformation. The truth is that if we go "all the way" to complete understanding in any aspect of our lives, we meet healing, wholeness, and holiness. I'm encouraging you to seize menopause as an opportunity to practice this whole-heart, whole-body, whole-mind stance in your life.

We can make change while continuing to crash along in our daily lives: "Yes, I'll file the divorce papers, have lunch with my friend Jane, and then stop at the nursery to pick up the cherry tree I ordered last week.. . ."

Without pausing, however, we cannot absorb the depth and richness of the moment. Change, when consciously undertaken, evokes *grace*.

Ceremony also offers our family and friends an opportunity to see and welcome us as different people. Women change going through menopause. We are different on the other side of this life transition, just as prepubescent girls are different from young women. Often menopausal women are more likely to say what they want to say, and do what they want to do. We need a circle of supporters who will welcome these changes and celebrate our newness.

This chapter is a primer for creating your own ritual to mark your menopausal transition. The tools presented here can also be applied to create rituals to mark other life passages, to pray, to invoke healing, to resolve grief, to let go of outdated patterns, and/or to begin a new chapter in your life.

SOLO JOURNEY, SOUL JOURNEY

Although the majority of this chapter focuses on creating a celebration with friends and family, an equally potent way of marking this life transition is a solo journey. Perhaps you have spent much of your life caring for others. You may have grown a business or nurtured a family. You may have gifted your community with many hours of devoted service. For you, the most powerful acknowledgment of your menopausal passage may be spending time alone.

Laura is a gregarious woman who pastors a Unity Church. As she approached her fiftieth birthday, she decided to celebrate in a completely new way. With more than a little trepidation, she booked a room on the Oregon coast for an entire week.

"I wasn't sure what to expect," she told me later. "I realized I had never been alone in my entire life." Her growing family and numerous church activities had consumed her attention and constantly kept her in contact with other people.

During her week on the coast, Laura took walks, read books, cooked meals, and wrote in her journal.

"The biggest surprise," she reported, "is that I like my own company."

You, too, may discover you are your own best companion. You may also discover that solitude nourishes you at least as deeply as communion with other people.

Walking the Sacred

I offer the following "Medicine Walk," based in part on the teachings of Dr. Beth Davis and Ruth Traut, as one example of a solo ceremony. In this context, "medicine" does not refer to aspirin or antibiotics, but rather a way of living that is healthy for body, mind, and spirit.

MEDITATION

Choose a day that has meaning for you—perhaps the one-year anniversary of your last menstrual period, full moon, new moon, or the death or birth of a beloved friend or family member. Clear your schedule. If you have children, arrange for someone else to care for them.

Call a friend before your journey, giving him or her the date and time you have planned your walk, and where you will be journeying. Let them know you plan to be home by a certain time, and that you will call them that evening before a certain hour. Prepare them ahead of time that you will just be checking in, not engaging in a long conversation, as you will want to remain in sacred space throughout the entire day.

Wake in the morning and take a ritual bath or shower. After dressing, smudge yourself with sage, sweetgrass, myrrh, or frankincense. Pack a water bottle and light food, if you plan to eat.

Walk or drive to the beginning place for your sacred walk. Choose a location where you are unlikely to be disturbed by other walkers or hikers, in as natural an environment as possible. You might choose a wilderness area or a local botanical garden. Offer prayers, and possibly tobacco or a special stone, asking that you be guided and blessed with wisdom as you walk.

Begin your walk, maintaining the open, relaxed attitude of "beginner's mind." Allow your attention to be drawn, your heart tugged, your mind tickled. Let yourself move and rest, dance and saunter as you are moved. Allow the earth to speak to you. Gently bend/apply your entire body to this task. Listen through your pores. Observe with your whole body, with every sense. All aspects of creation have the ability to "speak," but our minds need to be quiet enough, and our hearts receptive enough, to "hear" those communications. Take note of the events and encounters during the walk.

At the end of your journey, offer thanks. You might offer more tobacco, a prayer, and/or a song or insight that you received during the sacred walk.

When you arrive home, create a story in your journal describing your journey in the third person, for example, "Sara left an offering of home-baked bread at the Sunset Mesa trailhead. She sat for most of an hour watching the birds and chipmunks feasting on her offering. With slow steps, weighted by her hiking books, she began to climb the spine of the mesa. A flock of small birds Sara did not recognize alighted on a bush near the top of the mesa. Sara stopped to listen to their sociable twittering that reminded her so much of the chatter that filled the room when her menopausal friends' group, 'Compost in Bloom,' gathered. . . ."

Writing or telling a friend about your journey in the third person may spark insights that you may not have gleaned speaking in the first person "I." You gain a bit of distance and perspective from this storytelling stance. The journey has the opportunity to move beyond ordinary details to the realm of mythic patterns. What does the story have to tell you about what is happening in your life now, or in the future? Allow the specific details to coalesce into a larger shape, a more complex pattern.

Pay special attention to your encounters during the rest of the day, and your dreams that night. The wisdom you receive during the walk will likely continue to gestate in the rest of your life.

If you receive guidance, act on it. Creator knows you are serious, and often bestows more wisdom and guidance on those who are willing to enact it. Wisdom without action is impotent. Ideas can gather like clutter in our minds. If you receive inspiration about a project you know you will never enact, pass it on. Consciously let go of it by gifting it to someone else, or sending it back to the "Cosmic Pot."

Brooke Medicine Eagle reminds us that in the Grandmother Lodge, wisdom or inspiration may come specifically to pass on to others. Does any of your journey include gifts for others? Are you being reminded that you have wisdom or physical gifts to share with others?

When you return home, you may wish to prepare a celebratory meal, to eat alone or with others. Make a spirit plate (see below) to honor the seen and unseen beings who have assisted you on this medicine walk.

Ceremony for Right Relationship with Self and Others

You may choose to mark your menopausal transition in the company of others. At its heart, ceremony and ritual are intended to place us in good relationship with ourselves, our community, and the Divine. I have outlined the basic elements of ceremony: creating sacred space, raising energy, directing energy, and closing the space. Within this basic framework, you have lots of room for inspiration and improvisation.

Before you plan your celebration, clarify your intention. What are you celebrating? Will you focus on what has been, and/or what you are becoming? What do you want to invoke? Who do you want to become? How do you want to enter this next phase of your life? What will you take with you, and what will you discard?

Take time to reflect on these and other questions that may occur to you as you walk, journal, pray, or meditate. The effect of the ceremony can only be as powerful as the clarity of your intentions.

Creating Sacred Space

Sacred space is on the earth, but not of it. Consecrated territory becomes a portal for the Divine to enter our lives.

Sometimes a sacred space has obvious boundaries: the walls of a church or the skin of a sweat lodge. We can also create sacred space that is not visible to the casual observer. After such an area has been utilized in a ceremonial way for a long time, even the untrained, unaware observer will recognize something "different" about the space.

In Australia, aboriginal people have used certain ceremonial sites for over forty thousand years. White settlers, completely ignorant of aboriginal traditions, would sometimes stumble on these sites and run screaming from them, terrified by the "other-worldly" things they experienced there. The imprint of that sacred portal was so deeply imbued in the land that the place affected even the profoundly unaware.

I found many of these aboriginal sacred sites to be deeply peaceful places of healing. I was also fortunate to have support and guidance, as well as clear intention, in entering these sites.

To mark and create sacred space, you may want to incorporate one or more of the following suggestions:

- Create a circle with pinecones, rocks, shells, or other natural objects to mark sacred space. Choose biodegradable objects that can return to the soil after ceremony. If you use rocks, ask inwardly which rocks want to be moved to create this new space. Ask again after the ceremony if they want to stay or be returned to their original spot.

- Bless water and sprinkle it around the boundaries of your sacred space. If possible draw water from a spring or clean, running river. If desired, you can add a pinch of salt along with your intention for the ceremony. Hold the water and imbue it with your prayers. Water has extraordinary abilities to absorb our intentions. The preparation of homeopathic medicines is based on water's ability to carry the imprint of another substance. *The Hidden Messages in Water* by Masaru Emoto is also a testimony to water's ability to reflect intention.

- Walk several times around the ceremonial site, imprinting the earth with your intention for the ceremony. In Tibet and Nepal, this practice is known as "circumambulation." Walking around a sacred area activates the site and blesses the walker.

- Acknowledge the seven directions to prepare the site. From ancient Celtic traditions, I have learned to recognize rather than invoke the directions. I do not have to command or manipulate these massive energies. They surround me at all times. My job is to become aware of their presence and welcome them into the circle. The seven directions include East, South, West, North, Above, Below, and Within.

♦ If you are creating a solo ritual, you can mentally draw a circle or sphere around you. Imagine sitting in a huge tepee that rises above you, or resting in a cave in the center of a mountain. You can also envision a golden pyramid rising above you, with the central point above your head.

Cleansing

If you already have a place set aside for ceremony and ritual, you can prepare the space by "smudging" or other cleansing methods.

SMUDGING

Many native North American people burn sage, sweetgrass, cedar, and/or tobacco to prepare for ceremony. Western studies have demonstrated that burning sage, or "smudging," ionizes the air, literally changing the electro-magnetic environment. The censers in Catholic churches, filled with frank-incense, are another example of smudging. Studies of essential oils demonstrate that frankincense can profoundly affect brain chemistry[1], placing us in an altered state that supports spiritual opening.

MISTING

Mist the space with essential oils diluted in water. Keep in mind that essential oils are extremely concentrated and must be used respectfully. A drop of essential oil is equivalent to approximately thirty cups of tea. You will need to dilute essential oils (directions below) in order to use them safely. Some essential oils that are helpful for space clearing and are safe for children include lavender and rose. Other oils that are also helpful for cleansing but are *not* safe for use with children include all of the conifers (for example, spruce, fir, pine) and the citrus family (lemon, orange, tangerine, grapefruit).

Dilutions Create a $1/2$ to 1 percent dilution of essential oils in a spray bottle (ideally a glass spray bottle if you can find it, as essential oils will eventually destroy a plastic bottle). Avoid the eyes when you mist.

♦ 1 percent dilution: To eight ounces of water, add fifty drops of essential oil. Add one to two tablespoons vodka or other alcohol to disperse the essential oil in water.

- ◆ $1/2$ percent dilution: To eight ounces of water, add twenty-five drops of essential oil. Add one to two tablespoons vodka or other alcohol to disperse the essential oil in water.

Shake well before spraying.

Saltwater Mix salt into freshwater, offering prayers as you stir to dissolve the salt. Flick the saltwater around the space.

Self-cleansing You may choose to take a ceremonial bath before a ritual. See Molly Scott's interview (p. XXX) for inspiration in creating your own cleansing ritual.

Raise Energy

After learning how to create my own rituals, I was better able to appreciate the religious sacraments of my childhood. In the Methodist church, the early part of the service involves "raising energy." Hymns, music, responsive readings, and biblical readings are all part of focusing and stirring devotion in the congregation. Other churches, such as the Pentecostal and some Baptist churches, have much more passionate ways of stirring the congregation, with gospel singing, testimonials, and speaking in tongues.

For your passage ceremony, you may choose to sing hymns, chant, read poetry, dance, or play music together. Anything that stirs the soul, opens the heart, and focuses the mind is appropriate. If you are celebrating with a group, this part of the ritual also bonds the circle. Together you create a chalice to receive inspiration, wisdom, blessing, and healing.

Enact What You Want to Become

Within the sacred realm, you can enact or become what you want to be. If I want to receive abundance in my life, for example, I need to adopt a posture that signals receptivity. I might stand with my arms outstretched, my chest open and relaxed, to signal my preparedness to receive. I am training my mind and spirit through my body posture to adopt new patterns and habits. If my body remains contracted, my mind and spirit will also be unable to receive the gifts that surround me.

Consider how you want to enter this phase in your life. What gifts do you want to bring with you? What new experiences do you want to invoke? Imagine the qualities you want to embody.

With these images clearly in mind, ask how you could symbolically or actually enact those experiences in a ritual.

One woman entering a new phase in her life gathered friends and asked them to form a birthing canal. We stood in two lines, our palms facing into the canal. She spoke of her hopes and dreams for the life she was entering, and noted what aspects she was leaving behind. As she entered the "canal," we gently touched her body so she could physically experience her passage. She emerged laughing and crying, with tears streaming down her face. We offered gifts, prayers, and songs to welcome her into a new world.

Be creative. The enactment only needs to make sense to you and your body. Trust your body wisdom, your most ancient link to Source, to guide you.

Direct Energy, Offer Blessings

Now is the time to direct the divine energy you have invited and focused in your sacred space. If the circle is devoted to healing, for example, one of the circle participants might be placed in the center of the circle while other participants direct their prayers and blessings to that person. Blessings and prayers can also be directed to those not present.

In Blessing Way ceremonies, for mothers soon to give birth, celebrants bring beads to gift the expectant mother. Each bead is given with a prayer or blessing for the mother and baby-to-be. The mother strings the beads together and wears those prayers during labor and the early days of the child's life. Both mother and child draw upon the support of their family and community so simply and eloquently made visible through the strand of beads the mother wears.

For your ritual, consider how you would feel most comfortable being gifted by friends and family. You may also want the circle to devise this segment of the ritual for you. Make sure you have a "point person" responsible for this part of the ceremony, unless you are comfortable with complete spontaneity. You will likely know ahead of time, from previous experience, whether or not your circle of celebrants is able to move spontaneously, or whether they need more time to prepare.

Closing the Circle

♦ Most Native American ceremonies end with thanksgiving for all of creation. Without the support of every aspect of creation, our lives could not go on. We are strands in an enormously complex, interconnected web. You may choose to express your thanks by offering prayers, food, and/or song and music. Many native people make a "spirit plate" before eating a ceremonial meal. Someone places a small portion of each dish prepared for the celebration on a plate and leaves the plate outside as a "spirit offering." That food nourishes the local wildlife as well as the unseen spirits of ancestors, spirit helpers and spirit keepers, angels, guides—the host of "helpers" who assist us in so many (often unknown and unacknowledged) ways.

♦ In Asia, many people prepare a spirit plate daily, leaving it outside the back door for whomever wishes to partake. I loved frequenting a Thai restaurant in Portland, Oregon, where a beautifully arranged "spirit plate," with a stick of incense burning next to it, graced the local neighborhood. You may choose to make the spirit plate a daily ritual.

♦ Offer thanks to the directions for joining your celebration. You may choose to move around the circle, beginning in the East and progressing to the South, West, and North, then focusing Above, Below, and Within. Offer your appreciation to these presences in your life. They are witnessing and supporting your life transition.

♦ Be sure to close the circle in some fashion. You have invited a host of seen and unseen folk. Let them know when the "work" is complete.

♦ In the Christian church, this is called the "benediction," a final blessing on the congregation before they leave the church to resume their daily lives. "We are closing sacred space," says the minister/priest. "May the blessings of this time follow you into the rest of your life."

Sharing "Tea and Cakes"

After the formal closing of the circle, many traditions share food and drink. Among the ancient Celts, the offering was usually tea and sweet cakes. This food and drink "grounds" the physical body, reconnecting us with our physicality after journeying in the spirit realms. Eating and drinking also provides a forum for people to talk and share informally, which is an important aspect of strengthening personal and community bonds.

Creating Ceremony with a Group

Instead of focusing ceremony on an individual woman, a group may choose to celebrate life transitions together. Ruth Traut, a gifted ceremonialist and teacher, described the following ritual she cocreated with a group in Germany. The women met in a ritual space with lovely, quiet music playing in the room. Each woman was at a different stage of the life cycle, marking a major life change. They sat in a circle and talked about what they were leaving behind and what they were moving toward. In silence, the women drew images of what they were leaving behind, and then images of what they wanted to become. The circle met again, and the women shared their pictures.

The women then shed their clothes, down to underpants. The women painted each other with body paint, using the images each woman had described. On the back, they painted symbols of what that woman was leaving behind; on the front they painted what she was moving toward.

"This was a deep honoring of our bodies, all of our different shapes and sizes. We were honoring and decorating our bodies," explained Ruth.

There was a sweat lodge at the location where they were gathered, and the women used it "as the ceremonial womb that it is." Each woman moved by herself into the lodge, and spoke whatever she wanted to about what she was leaving behind and what she moving toward. The women rotated positions. As a woman emerged from the sweat lodge, two other women helped wash the images from her back, removing what she was leaving behind. Each woman chose when she wanted to remove the images on her front.

After this ritual washing, the woman moved to a bench where she had left special ceremonial garb. Two women waiting at the bench helped dress her. Then she in turn helped the women emerging from the lodge. The women rotated positions throughout the ritual.

"There was very little verbal communication in the ritual," says Ruth. "The entire ceremony, both the processing and the enacting, was almost completely nonverbal. Some of the women had a hard time with that, but I think the silence allowed us to move into a very deep, transformative space. The ceremony was simple, and quite lovely."

PLANTING THE SEED

The ritual you have created is a beginning, the onset of a new journey, the altering of the course of the river. The ritual plants a seed, and you water it with your actions. As you continue to tend that seed, *feel* as well as see the embodiment of your vision. Seeing and feeling together are powerful fertilizers for your seedling. Seeing alone will not yield the results you want.

Solo rituals are powerful. The gathering of friends and family can be even more potent because those community members augment the power of your own vision by adding their own focused concentration on its manifestation. Of course they can't do the tending work for you, the actual physical labor, but they can *see* you in your new form. They help hold the blueprint, like the devic pattern, to assist you in growing into a new form.

Reflections by Molly Scott

As a musician, performer, and recording artist, Molly Scott has devoted her performing and songwriting career to supporting issues of peace and social justice. As a therapist and educator, Dr. Scott has focused her clinical work and research on the role that vocal resonance plays in the healing process, particularly in the treatment of trauma. A pioneer in the use of the voice in therapy, Molly Scott began to develop her healing work with the voice as a young singer when she became curious about the effect her own voice had upon her feelings and her health. She began leading groups in the 1970s and has expanded her work with the voice and healing into a therapeutic model called Creative Resonance, which she has been teaching for more than twenty years in the United States, Canada, and Europe. She is the director of the Creative Resonance Institute, which offers trainings in the use of voice for healing professionals. She works with singers, musicians, and writers in heightening creativity and performance and presentation skills, and she started the musical group, "Sumitra." She teaches counseling at Antioch New England Graduate School in Keene, N.H, has a private practice in Shelburne Falls and Charlemont, MA and is on staff with the MSPCC Family Counseling Center in Greenfield, MA. Her poems have appeared in several journals, and she is working on a collection of her poetry and a book on the role of voice in therapy.

I started menopause in my mid- to late-forties. The physical changes were not so difficult; the psychic ones were. It was a time of soul-searing reassessment, starting several years before my fiftieth birthday and continuing for several years after. Looking back now from the vantage of almost twenty years, I reflect that what brought me through the difficulties was a sense of community with other women across time that was deeper than my conscious knowing—an understanding that this process moving in me was as profound as giving birth was and as death may be. Despite the darkly negative picture contemporary culture painted of menopause and the juiceless hagdom waiting on the other side, I felt something powerful happening in my soul and spirit as well as my body, and I was determined to rise to meet it.

My immediate family offered no models: my mother had had a hysterectomy in her thirties and didn't speak about her hormonal changes with her two daughters, and my grandmother, who seemed always to have been old, would have been shocked to have menopause mentioned in "polite conversation." Indeed, there *was* nothing polite about menopause: too much blood or too little, too much sweat, and more tears than most of us would want to admit.

Lacking familial models, I invoked mythic ones. Although I grew up in little-town

America, I derived a rich sense of Celtic lineage from my family background—Scots and Scots-Irish on both sides of my family. As a child, I was steeped in the tradition of the highland bards and warriors, the storytellers and magic makers in a time and place where aging was honored and the triple goddess—maiden/mother/crone—reigned over the western islands and the ancient world everywhere.

I also looked to the goddess mythology from the Greco-Roman world for mentors and models: Persephone, queen of the underworld, and her earth mother, Demeter, and most of all the fierce figure of Hecate, the wise-woman crone.

Rescuing the Crone

The idea of the crone as a positive, generative force has been degraded in Western culture. Magnificent Hecate, she who stands at the crossroad, guarding our birthing and our dying, has been reduced to the hag, the purveyor of evil magic, the witch. This denigration has reduced the power and beauty of aging into cultural invisibility.

I had met the feminine three-in-one in the Celtic world, traveling in Ireland and Scotland. In one aspect, she was known as Brige, Bridie, Bridghid of the healing wells, and I had sung to her, hanging clootie prayer rags over her miraculous springs. In old stone sites, and even, surprisingly, in monasteries and cloisters, I had seen ferocious carved images of the Sheela Na Gig with her gaping vagina-mouth birthing the world. I had also met her in India as the dark side of radiant tiger-riding Durga—terrifying Kali, with skulls and bodies dripping from her bloody mouth. In my Buddhist practice, she was present in the Vajra Yogini, the Great Bliss Queen, powerful Sky Woman who embodied primordial wisdom, "unfabricated, natural, self-arising."

There was nothing like this in the white-bread Christianity in which I was raised. The powerful matriarch, the "wise, willful, wolfish crone"[2] as Barbara Walker called her in her book Crone, had been defanged into Mary Mother Mild. These images from other cultures, other times, were both alluring and appalling to me. How could I relate to this? How could I leave the Barbie doll expectations of my upbringing and cross into this landscape of wild, powerful, idiosyncratic women, aging and ageless? And how could I *not*?

Later, joining with other women as part of the woman's movement, in ritual circles and in political actions like the women's peace camps, my image of "woman" began to change. Through my own experiences, I had been reworking my ideas and feelings about what it is to be a woman. I saw women—focused, energetic, empowered women of all ages, sizes, and ethnicities—working together for a greater vision than the limited roles to which we had been assigned.

Life Hinges

My menopause served as a hinge between distinct periods of my life which, like maiden/mother/crone, seem to have three phases. As the marriage ceremony traditionally marked the hinge between the child and the adult—in earlier times, occurring as the menses came and the child was able to bear children—so menopause is the biological hinge between the adult and the elder. Although the Protestant culture in which I had been raised lacked a cultural marker, such markers do exist. In Judiasm, there is the ceremony of *simhat hochmah*, a celebration of grandmother or crone wisdom, and many indigenous societies have rituals that consecrate menopause as a time when the blood of creative life force, no longer expressed as children, stays within the woman and becomes Wisdom. I felt the need for some outward ceremony to mark this inner passage into the third phase of my life and so I determined to create one.

I had married, for the first time, in my twenties, with all the accoutrements of the cultural passage (good food, great party), but little of spiritual commitment that marks deep change. The real rite of passage for me came with the birth of my first child, a daughter. Holding her for the first time, a luminous space opened in me in which I ceased to be a child and became a Mother. The change went deep in my bones, and the world changed around it like a sounding bell.

In retrospect, menopause was like that as well—a change so incontrovertible that the landscape on one side bore little resemblance to that on the other. However, this passage into the third phase of my life, from mother to elder/crone, has happened in a long, slow arc—and is still happening. The croning ceremony I created served as a signifier for layers of meaning that continue to unfold across time. Now I am birthing myself, and it may take until my dying to be fully born. Perhaps that *is* what dying is . . .the final birthing of the Self into a changed reality.

My fiftieth birthday fell in the middle of this time, and it became the opportunity to create ritual that both marked and assisted the changes I felt and the shift I longed for. I wanted to create a ritual that would consecrate passage into the third phase, a ceremony that would signal *Conjunctio,* the sacred marriage of the self to the Self. I knew the power of ritual. I'd been leading groups in sound and healing in the United States and Europe for many years, had created ceremonies in ancient sites all over the world, and had developed a repertoire of tools to assist others in transformational change. Now I wanted to participate in my own ceremony of crossing. I wanted to gather a circle of love around me, a gathering of friends and family to help spark, kindle, and burn change into this next part of my life.

Making Ceremony, Making Meaning

The plan was that people would come to my home, share a meal, and participate in the ceremony. Sharing food was an important element of the environment upon which this plan was built. In our rural community, the occasional potluck gathering lets us know, across the distance between us, that we are still here for each other. Music was also integral—music for me to sing and music to sing together. I was well known in the community as a singer, and many of my songs had choruses that people knew. I was clear that this event was not to be a performance but a ceremony in which music was used as part of the process. Although there were several songs I wanted to sing, like "Centering Home," which had been a signature journey song for me for many years, I also wanted to leave space for what arose in the moment.

The alchemical core of the ceremony, the catalyst in the alembic of the sacred circle, was that I would speak and sing the story of my life, with my friends and family serving as the energetic container in which the story could be witnessed, experienced, and charged to change. My intention was to transit through the difficult, shadowed places in my past as best I could in order to move beyond them. I wanted to invoke the qualities, and energetic models, that would in-form the next part of my life, as my daughter said, "Your next fifty years."

The Ceremony, like the stages of my life, was in three stages: the Preparation, the Passage, and the Transformation.   Here's what happened.

The Preparation

In early afternoon, a small group of women came to massage, bathe, and prepare me for the evening event. There were nine: my daughter, my sister and her daughter, my son's new Dutch girlfriend who later became my daughter-in-law, and a few close friends. They gently removed my clothes and softly put their hands on me, oiling, massaging, and speaking about my body and who I was to them. My daughter was twenty, in early womanhood, and she rose to this ceremony, taking a strong role. She and my friends acknowledged that this body of mine was both beautiful and aging, and that this process is natural and good. We read passages about Old Woman, creator of the world, from Anne Cameron's lovely book *Daughters of Copper Woman*,[3] which many of us were reading at the time. There is a better way of doing things. Some of us remember that better way," the storyteller said, and we were mindful that our ceremony was a kind of remembering and moving to that ancient way.

This was my first challenge, early in the process, to let myself receive this loving touch and these stories without feeling self-conscious about my body or that I needed to give back. My learning was to allow, and to receive, with the understanding that to deeply receive is a gift to the giver.

I was deeply moved by this process. In the massage and the bath that followed, the stories the women told took on an everywoman cast: how this was the body of a baby who became a little girl who became a woman. How this woman became a mother, how this mother body grew a daughter and a son. My daughter witnessed my body as the place from which she had come, and she acknowledged that her own body might also birth children, perhaps a granddaughter for me, continuing the line of the family women. (Indeed, this has happened; she gave birth to a daughter in a warm-water birthing tub with her partner, fifteen other women, and me in rapt attendance. I saw my granddaughter crown in my daughter's body, like the Sheela Na Gig, and rise to the surface looking at everyone with wide-open eyes as I sang "Amazing Grace.")

After the bath, the women toweled, dressed me, and handed me my "staff"—a shepherd's crook that I had brought back from Scotland with great difficulty on the airplane (I kept hooking people and saying, "Sorry, sorry!"). A seamstress friend had pieced together some of my favorite old clothes to make a high-collared robe, multicolored and patched together, like my life. I wore it over a black top and pants with pockets. The pockets were important; they held a pen to write things during the ceremony, a capo for my guitar, and lots of tissue in case I cried. I did.

The Passage: Setting It Up

As dusk fell, the rest of the guests arrived—including my son, my partner, and the partners of the other women—bundled in winter gear, stamping and blowing from the cold, bringing food and small gifts. (My son later told me that the family men felt "banished" from the afternoon events, something I would want to reconsider were I to do it again.) I had set up my vaulted living room so that people could sit in a half circle around me. My small grand piano was behind me and several guitars so that I could play and sing if I was moved to do so. A little table covered with a paisley cloth served as an altar. The woodstove was cooking away in the corner keeping the cold away, and various dogs, cats, and babies were splayed about on rug, couches, and laps. The people, the musical instruments, and the altar made the circle.

After the shared meal I welcomed people and explained the idea behind this gathering. I said that it was a time of transition in my life and I was asking for the energetic lift of their stories, thoughts, and blessings to carry me through to another place—the other side of fifty and whatever it might hold. I asked them to join me in a song to start our tuning in together. We sang "Centering Home," a song I wrote in 1970 with a simple, singable chorus:

Walking along, hearing the words
that the people are saying
sensing the circular plans we're laying
knowing that I will be
part of the things I see...

People joined in on the chorus, my two grown children, my sister, nieces and nephew, all wonderful singers, adding harmony:

Strange how my feet keep walking
no other path but this path
strange how my heart keeps saying
no other words but these words
Home...Centering home, Centering home, Centering home...[4]

Passage: A Ceremonial Marriage of Self to Self

I turned to the altar then, where there were three bowls or vessels in front of me along with three candles representing past, present, and future. The first vessel was a small metal caldron, for burning those things from my past that I no longer wished to carry forward. The second vessel, another bowl, was for saving those qualities I wanted to carry forward with me into the future. The third vessel, a clear glass bowl filled with water, was for transmutation, a place to put visions and dreams, my own and others', energizing them in water so they could continue to flow into my life. I had asked guests to bring a special stone or crystal to add to the water in the ceremony with prayers and blessings for me, the earth, and each other. I lit each candle as I moved from bowl to bowl until the little altar was glowing with fire.

Passage: Reworking the Myth of Molly

Now came the heart of the ritual, in which I alternately spoke, sang, and sounded my way through the highs and lows of my life story. It was daunting. I had been through some difficult times in my life and didn't know if I had words for what I wanted to release. I resolved that if I couldn't speak something easily, I would sing it, knowing that singing changes the brain waves and that I would then perceive what I was singing about differently.

If there were no words to express what I needed to convey, I gave myself the option of using what I called nonlanguage sounding, NLS, or gibberish, to keep my emotional energy flowing without getting stuck in descriptive language. I learned this technique during my early theater training, using gibberish as a way to stay with an emotion without getting caught in text. I've since found this method, which I call Deep Story, useful in the treatment of trauma, when words are inadequate to the experience, or there are no words at all. In the ceremony, the opportunity to express emotional memory without revealing content also gave me a safety valve to keep elements of my story private if need be but to still feel and experience them without words impeding the core movement of the process.

Maintaining privacy of content was important for another reason. My elderly mother, just on the edge of Alzheimer's, was there, and, just as I knew that involving her in earlier preparation would have been much too "touchy-feely" for her (not to mention the nudity!), I was aware that too much truth telling might stress and confound her. "Not my generation's thing," she would say. But I wanted and needed her to be there with me to share the experience at whatever level she could. I remember standing by the altar, starting to tell my birth story which, of course, began with her, looking over at her where she sat in a chair near the woodstove. She looked back at me with her very blue eyes, and in that moment, I *understood* in a way that I never quite had before, that I had come out of this woman's living body as my daughter and son had emerged from mine.

I was formed from her blood and juices, from her love and intention. I asked her to tell us what she remembered of my birth, and she did, the old wheels of memory creaking back. I honored her then, and asked the circle to honor her also, and their own mothers.

Passage: Transmutation

And so it went. I explored and exploded my way through my story, laughing, sometimes crying, singing here and there, putting strips of paper in the Burn Bowl and some in the Keep Bowl. I burned *taking responsibility for that unnamed grief in the place where people wept and the shades were drawn.* I did this "in tongues," meaning NLS or gibberish. I also burned *the greed of holding on* and a story about a childhood friend. And I put into the fire *the pain, the adolescent tangle of not knowing who I was—the power, passion, and angst of growing up in an alien environment. I leave it. I am not bound by it anymore.* I asked people in the circle to hum while I did this, in order to create the resonant field, and so that they could also feel part of this intensely personal process they were witnessing.

I remember how exposed I felt during this part of the ritual, particularly during the nonlanguage sounding, how scary it was, but also how necessary. I was ready for it, as one is ready to dive into cold water on a hot day, yet still hesitates, anticipating the shock.

The next day in my journal I made of list of What I Kept: *Memories of deep green lake, morning daffodils, hillsides in afternoon sun, nights in gardens with blue flowers in the dark; playing the piano by moonlight when everyone is asleep. (The moon taught me to play the piano.)*

And I made affirmations from the What I Kept: *My children are my teachers; I trust what is coming towards me on the other side of menopause; I have faith in the continuing abundance of my life.*

Passage Through: Transmutation in Community

For the last part of the ceremony, I moved to the third bowl, the large transparent glass one, filled with water. It was time then for other people to speak and share stories, and to come up to the altar and gift their prayers and blessings into the water. The concept was that these energies would be transmuted into the water, which would then be charged with them. Now, almost twenty years later, with the work of Dr. Masaru Emoto[5] we know that the crystalline structure of water does indeed change with the subtle energies of thought, giving credence to my intention in this ceremony that the water would receive and transmit the prayers and blessings of the participants. Some people put in little stones or crystals that they had brought and said things out loud. Other people just came up and hugged me in silence.

Closing the ceremony with this ritual provided a way of ending that expanded our circle beyond the little house in the woods and my little life, and beyond our small rural community, and out to the world. We invoked the richness of the earth, the goodness in the turn of the seasons, the blessings of the surrounding forest and the great, resonant Family of Things. We ended by singing my song "We Are All One Planet."

We are all one planet,
All one people of earth
All one planet,
sharing our living, our dying, our birth
and we won't stand by
watching her die,
hearing her cry and deny
we live as she lives,
  we die as she dies.[6]

Then people gathered dishes, coats, babies, and each other and went back into the night.

I had intended to spend the rest of the night in meditation in my tower, but reality kicked in and I fell into bed, exhausted, satisfied, sated with stories and ritual doings, and slept soundly into the next morning. I woke into New Time. I was fifty-one, half the way through menopause, and perhaps only halfway through my long and wonderful life.

Coda

My life did indeed change on the other side of that Birthday ritual. Within a year I had entered a graduate program for what I thought would be a three-year degree but which stretched to eight as I went on to complete my doctorate in Consulting Psychology. Going back to school, a whole world opened to me, full of surprises. One was that I fell in love with science and took courses I would not have considered in my undergraduate years. Another was that that the skills I had cultivated as a singer, performer, composer, and workshop leader had value in the world of psychotherapy. I discovered that I was a natural counselor. Indeed, in some sense, it was what I had been doing all along.

And I can say, unequivocally, that on this side of menopause, the energy of my life is markedly different. I am less troubled, much happier. Whereas before, the graph of my life went up and down in monthly peaks and valleys, now I experience the flow of my energy as smooth and constant. I see myself in those earlier years as more caught up in surface weather, buffeted by winds, surprised by sudden squalls. Often I thought that I sailed alone through my storms of troubles and that my boat was fragile and small.

That, too, has shifted. I have the experience daily of living as part of an interwoven community of life: wind, tree, cat, horse, dog, flower. When I remember to center and be present with the open ears of my heart, I know that I am not alone. Life has gifted me with a friendlier, more luminous inner weather. Of course, it is not always as neat as that. My life has not been free of troubles or without devastating surprises, but who I am has truly shifted over time and I am no longer so blown off course by small things.

Molly can be reached at: Creative Resonance Institute, 327 Warner Hill, Charlemont, MA 01339; 413-339-5501; Fax 413-339-0144; mollyscott@mollyscott.com

Please visit: www.mollyscott.com
www.creativeresonance.com

www.sumitrafoundation.com
www.sumitra.org

Poem by Caitlín Matthews

Caitlín Matthews is a respected initiator in the Shamanic, Celtic and Arthurian traditions, and she has opened many doors to a reappreciation of the mythic heritage of the Western World. She and her husband, John, are the authors of over ninety books, which have translated into French, Italian, Spanish, German, Czech, Dutch, Hebrew, Portuguese, Danish, Korean, Japanese, Finish and Russian. Caitlín's books include The Da Vinci Enigma Tarot, Celtic Devotional, *and* Sophia, Goddess of Wisdom, Bride of God.

I wrote this poem in the last phase of menopause—a threnody and prophecy both that explores the strange fragmentation of meaning as menopause strikes. It is about finding the rhythm of creativity when the priorities are in a state of alteration.

I personally don't feel I have become a crone—that will happen when my bits start to drop off. There is a phase between mother and crone that happens when we become the protectors, actively involved in our community—guides of the tribe perhaps. I'm not ready for the rocking chair yet by a long chalk! While I have my own teeth, I intend to bite life's crust with relish.

Menopause

They pass, the bright dancers, down the long path of blood,
Leaving an empty story and a kicked-off shoe on the sod.
There's only a drift of music through the daily market's cry
And a long regret that impeaches the innocent Lenten sky.

Each of the dancing partners who swung me in their sway
Have passed like smoke from a hearthfire on a burning summer's day.
The passionate feet that bore me now dance to a different tune,
The love that was bright between us, turns dark as the changing
moon.

I search for the shards of story upon a jagged shore,
As Isis in her mourning sought for the scattered lore.
Only the plaintive curlew its solitary fluting makes
As over the barren hillside an empty morning breaks.

The hollow daylight departing, I lift my pleading eyes,
And out of the gentle darkness, see destiny's star arise.
Down its shimmering pathway, the ancient promises ride,
A hope that the dancing had blinded, a sure and certain guide.

A melody pure and perfect, a song from the heart of time,
Reverberates the darkness, making the dead boughs chime.
Fruit sets on the fruitless branches as stars come tumbling out,
An untold story dances on the shivering shores of doubt.

Caitlín can be reached at: BCM Hallowquest, London WC1N 3XX, U.K.

Epilogue

"Mine your spirit for the source of all treasure."

River Woman's hand sweeps forward, taking in the expanse of ocean.

"What treasure could be more magnificent, more valuable, more nourishing than the ocean? This watery expanse is the primary source of life on this planet. We carry the ocean in our blood, tears, and vaginal secretions. We carry this sea of life within us.

"We also carry spirit within us. I'm not talking about being a demi-God, invincible and unaccountable for all you do. No, just as you carry a cup of the ocean's magnificence within you, so also do you carry an echo of spirit within you. Creator lives and breathes through you, yet you are not Creator. The ocean moves within you, nourishing every cell, yet you are not the ocean. Do you understand?"

I nod quietly.

"And you are in me, River Woman."

She smiles.

"Your voice rings in my soul," I murmur. "Your thoughts touch my own."

"Yes, in truth each soul who is similarly attuned rings, or vibrates. We hum sympathetically, like the piano wire that resonates with a singer's voice or a child's squeal of delight. We touch one another with thoughts and feelings."

River Woman faces the ocean, her elbows resting on her bent knees, her hands clasped before her.

"The journey is only beginning," she reminds me. "You've broken down to pure elements so that you can re-form yourself at this time in your life. Set your course. Gather your provisions—a clear mind, a wise heart, and a penetrating soul. This food will carry you long after your legs have failed and your water bottle has run dry. Walk with spirit. Bring heaven into earth with each footstep. Bring earth to heaven with each thought.

"Keep me you in your heart. The river always flows down to the sea. You will never be lost."

APPENDIX

CHARTS

Any text here?

Diet Diary for _____ Beginning Date _____

The purpose of this diary is to provide you and your doctor with an unbiased record of your normal eating habits. Simply eat your typical diet and record what you eat for seven days in succession. Under breakfast, lunch, and dinner columns list food and drink ingredients and amounts. Under BM, list bowel movement times. Under Notes, list symptoms such as mood swings, indigestion, headaches, fatigue, and so on. Remember to include snacks and supplements (brand name, ingredients, potency).

	SUNDAY	MONDAY	TUESDAY	WEDNESDAY	THURSDAY	FRIDAY	SATURDAY
BREAKFAST							
LUNCH							
DINNER							
BM TIMES							

Additional Notes:

Exercise Journal for _____ Beginning Date _____

The purpose of this diary is to provide you and your doctor with an unbiased record of your normal exercise habits. Simply follow your typical exercise routine and record what you do for seven days in sucession. For every day list the amount and type of exercise you do.

* Note any physical, mental, or emotional responses to exercise, such as muscle strains after certain kinds of exercise, enjoyment or dislike of particular types of exercise, and so on.

	SUNDAY	MONDAY	TUESDAY	WEDNESDAY	THURSDAY	FRIDAY	SATURDAY
AEROBIC							
STRENGTH-BUILDING							
STRETCHING							
ACTIVITIES OF DAILY LIVING							
RESPONSES TO EXERCISE*							

Additional Notes:

NOTES

CHAPTER 1—PREPARATION FOR THE JOURNEY

1. Martin, M. C., et al. 1993. Menopause without symptoms: The endocrinology of menopause among rural Mayan Indians. *American Journal of Obstetrics & Gynecology* 168:1839–45.

2. Hammar, M., et al. 1990. Does physical exercise influence the frequency of post-menopausal hot flushes? *Acta Obstet Gynecol Scand* 69:409–12.

3. Clorfene-Casten, Liane. 1996. *Breast Cancer: Poisons, Profits and Prevention.* Monroe, ME: Common Courage Press, 34.

4. ———. 33.

5. Reynolds, F. 1995. Suffering in silence: Women's experience of menopausal hot flushes. (Paper presented to the British Psychological Society's Annual Conference, March 1995). Reported in *The Mind and Menopausal Hot Flashes, Mental Med Update* 4(3):1–2.

6. Hunter, M. S., and K. L. M. Liao. 1995. Evaluation of a 4-session cognitive behavioral intervention for menopausal hot flashes (Paper presented to the British Psychological Society's Annual Conference, March 1995). Reported in The Mind and Menopausal Hot Flashes, *Mental Med Update* 4(3):1–2.

CHAPTER 2—CHART YOUR COURSE:
CREATING YOUR PERSONAL VISION OF HEALTH

1. Robert Fritz. *The Path of Least Resistance.* New York: Fawcett Columbine, 1984, 1989.

2. Essi Systems. 1991 *The Stress Map.* New York: Newmarket Press. To order, call 800-233-4830.

CHAPTER 3—HORMONAL CYCLES:
ROOTED IN THE WHEEL OF LIFE

1. Levi F., F. Lucchini, et al. 1996. Oral contraceptives, menopausal hormone replacement treatment and breast cancer risk. *Eur J Cancer Prev* 5(4):259–66.

2. Brinton, L. A., D. R. Brogan, et al. 1998. Breast cancer risk among women under 55 years of age by joint effects of usage of oral contraceptives and hormone replacement therapy. *Menopause* 5(3):145–51.

3. Chang, K. J., et al. 1995. Influences of percutaneous administration of estradiol and progesterone on human breast epithelial cell cycle in vivo. *Fertility and Sterility* 63(4).

4. Gambrell, Jr., R. D. 1987. Use of progestogen therapy. *American Journal of Obstetrics and Gynecology* 156:1304–13.

5. Cowan, L. D., L. Gordis, J. A. Tonascia, et al. 1981. Breast cancer incidence in women with a history of progesterone deficiency. *American Journal of Epidemiology* 114:209.

6. Schairer, C., J. Lubin, et al. 2000. Menopausal estrogen and estrogen-progestin replacement therapy and breast cancer risk. *JAMA* 283(4):485–91.

7. Ross, R. K., A. Paganini-Hill, et al. 2000. Effect of hormone replacement therapy on breast cancer risk: Estrogen versus estrogen plus progestin. *J Natl Cancer Inst* 92(4):328–32.

8. Koenig, H. L., M. Schumacher, et al. 1995. Progesterone synthesis and myelin formation by Schwann cells. *Science* 268(5216):1500–1503.

9. Chan, R. J., et al. 1998. Glucocorticoids and progestins signal the initiation and enhance the rate of myelin formation. *Proc Natl Acad Sci USA* 95(18):10459–64.

10. Thompson, M. A., and M. D. Adelson. 1993. Aging and development of ovarian epithelial carcinoma: the relevance of changes in ovarian stromal androgen production. *Advances in Experimental Medicine & Biology* 330:155–65.

11. Stepan, J. J., et al. 1989. Castrated men exhibit bone loss: effect of calcitonin treatment on biochemical indices of bone modeling. *Journal Clinical Endocrinological Metabolism* 69:523–27.

12. Savvas, M., J. W. Studd, et al. 1992. Increase in bone mass after one year of percutaneous oestradiol and testosterone implants in post-menopausal women who have previously received long-term oral oestrogens. *British Journal of Obstetrics & Gynaecology* 99(9):757–60.

13. Prior, MD, Jerilyn. 1998. Perimenopause—the ovary's frustrating grand finale. *A Friend Indeed* 14(7):1.

CHAPTER 4—HORMONES:
MESSENGERS OF BIOLOGY, MESSAGES FROM SPIRIT

1. Schairer, C., J. Lubin, et al. 2000. Menopausal estrogen and estrogen-progestin replacement therapy and breast cancer risk. *JAMA* 283(4):485–91.

2. Ross, R. K., A. Paganini-Hill, et al. 2000. Effect of hormone replacement therapy on breast cancer risk: Estrogen versus estrogen plus progestin. *J Natl Cancer Inst* 92(4):328–32; Crane, M.G. 1968. Discussion in *Metabolic Effects of Gonadal Hormones and Contraceptive Steroids.* New York: Plenum Press, p. 736.

3. Landau, R. L., and K. Lugibihl. 1961. The catabolic and natriuretic effects of progesterone in man. *Recent Prog. Horm. Res.* 17:249–81.

4. [Author's/editor's name needed.] 1996. Prudence and the Pill. *Harvard Women's Health Watch* 3(8):1.

5. Chang, K. J., et al. 1995. Influences of percutaneous administration of estradiol and progesterone on human breast epithelial cell cycle in vivo. *Fertility and Sterility* 63(4):785–91.

6. Gambrell, Jr., R. D. 1987. Use of progestogen therapy. *American Journal of Obstetrics and Gynecology* 156:1304-13.

7. Wright, Jonathon. 1978. *Natural Hormone Replacement Therapy*. [We need publisher location and name]

8. Reported in Follingstad, A. H. 1978. Estriol, the forgotten estrogen? *JAMA* 239(1):29–30.

9. Bulbrook R. D., M. C. Swain, D. Y. Wang, et al. 1976. Breast cancer in Britain and Japan: Plasma oestradiol-17ß, oestrone and progesterone and their urinary metabolites in normal British and Japanese women. *Eur J Cancer* 12:725–35.

10. Reported in Follingstad, A. H. 1978. Estriol, the forgotten estrogen? *JAMA* 239(1):29–30.

11. 1994. Update: Tamoxifen on trial. *Ms.* July/August. 21.

12. Dick, I. M., R. L. Prince, J. J. Kelly, and K. K. Ho. 1995. Oestrogen effects on calcitriol levels in post-menopausal women: A comparison of oral versus transdermal administration. *Clinical Endocrinology* 43(2): 219-24.

13. Sener, A.B., et al. 1996. The effects of hormone replacement therapy on uterine fibroids in postmenopausal women. *Fertility and Sterility* 65(2):354–57.

14. Kimzey, L. M., et al. 1991. Absorption of micronized progesterone from a nonliquifying vaginal cream. *Fertility and Sterility* 56:995–96.

15. Hudson, T. 1995 (June). Estrogen replacement therapy: A guide to conventional and "quasi-natural choices." *Townsend Letter for Doctors*, pp. 164–65.

16. ****

17. Estes, Clarissa Pinkola. *The Faithful Gardener: A Wise Tale About That Which Can Never Die.* San Francisco: HarperSanFrancisco, 1995. 74–75.

18. Hendricks, Gay, and Philip Johncock, eds. *Already Home: Radiant Wisdom and Life-Changing Meditations from Ramana Maharshi, Sri Nisargadatt, and Teachers of the Advaita Tradition.* Carlsbad, CA: Hay House, 2006. 28–29.

CHAPTER 5—PHYTOESTROGENS:
HERBAL KNOWLEDGE AND HEALING WISDOM

1. Hudson, Tori. 1999. *Women's Encyclopedia of Natural Medicine.* Los Angeles: Keats Publishing, p. 154.

2. Matthews, K., et al. 1989. Menopause and risk factors for coronary heart disease. *N Engl J Med* 321:641.

3. Adlercreutz, H., et al. 1991. Urinary excretion of lignans and isoflavonoid phytoestrogens in Japanese men and women consuming traditional Japanese diet. *Am J Clin Nutr* 54:1093–1100.

4. Eden, J., et al. 1994/1995. Hormonal effects of isoflavones (abstract). First International Symposium on the Role of Soy in Preventing and Treating Chronic Diseases: Proceedings from a symposium in Mesa, Arizona, on February 20–23, 1994. Published in *J Nutr* 125 (Suppl 3S):567S–808S.

5. Harding, C., et al. Dietary soy supplementation is oestrogenic in menopausal women (poster abstract). See Ref. 4, p. 46.

6. Anderson, F., et al. 1995. Meta-analysis of the effects of soy protein intake on serum lipids. *N Engl J Med* 333(5):276–82.

7. Bahram, H., et al. 1996. Dietary soybean protein prevents bone loss in an ovariectomized rat model of osteoporosis. *J Nutr* 126:161–67.

8. Nomura, A., et al. 1978. Breast cancer and diet among the Japanese in Hawaii. *Am J Clin Nutr* 31:2020–25.

9. Hirayama, T. 1986. A large-scale cohort study on cancer risks by diet—with special reference to the risk of reducing effects of green-yellow vegetable consumption. In Hayashi, Y., et al. *Diet, Nutrition and Cancer.* Tokyo: Japanese Scientific Society Press, pp. 41–53.

10. Lee, T., et al. 1991. Dietary effects on breast cancer risk in Singapore. *Lancet* 337:1197–1200.

11. Parkin, D., et al. 1992. Cancer incidence in five continents. Lyon: International Agency for Research on Cancer Scientific Publications No. 120; 6:301-431, 486–509.

12. Goodman, M., et al. 1997. Association of soy and fiber consumption with the risk of endometrial cancer. *Am J Epid* 146(4):294–306.

13. Aldercreutz, H. 1984. Does fiber-rich food containing animal lignan precursors protect against both colon and breast cancer? An extension of the fiber hypothesis. *Gastroent* 86:761–66.

14. Setchell, K., et al. Mammalian lignans and phytoestrogens: Recent studies on their formation, metabolism and biological role in health and disease. In Rowland, I. (ed.) 1988. *Role of the gut flora in toxicity and cancer.* London: Academic, pp. 315–45.

15. Hartwell, J. 1976. Types of anticancer agents isolated from plants. *Canc Treat Rep* 60:1031–67.

16. Macrae, W., et al. 1984. Biological activities of lignans. *Phytochem* 23:1207–20.

17. Duker, E. M., et al. 1991. Effects of extracts from *Cimicifuga racemosa* on gonadotropin release in menopausal women and ovariectomized rats. *Planta Medica* 57:420–24.

18. Li, M.X., et al. 1996/1997. Effects of *Cimicifuga rhizome* on serum calcium and phosphate levels in low calcium dietary rats and on bone mineral density in ovariectomized rats. *Phytomedicine* 3(4):379–85.

19. Warnock, G. 1985. Influencing menopausal symptoms with a phytotherapeutic agent. *Med Welt* 36:871–74.

20. Hirata, J., et al. 1997. Does dong quai have estrogenic effects in postmenopausal women? A double-blind, placebo-controlled trial. *Fertil Steril* 68(6):981–86.

21. D'Angelo, L. et al. 1986. A double-blind, placebo-controlled clinical study on the effect of a standardized ginseng extract on psychomotor performance in healthy volunteers. *J Ethnopharmacol* 16:15–22.

22. Bombardelli, E., et al. 1980. The effect of acute and chronic (Panax) ginseng saponins treatment on adrenal function; biochemical and pharmacological. Proceedings of the Third International Ginseng Symposium—Korean Ginseng Research Institute, pp. 9–16.

23. Punnonen, R., et al. 1980. Oestrogenlike effect of ginseng. *Br Med J* 281:1110.

CHAPTER 6—THE SCIENCE OF TRANSFORMATION: EXTERNAL AND INTERNAL LANDSCAPES

1. Kos, Kala H., and John Selby. *The Power of Aloha*. www.hawaiiheart.com/hu'na.html.

2. Rumi

3. Pintar, Judith. 1996. *A Voice from the Earth: The Cards of Winds and Changes*. Stamford, CT: United States Games Systems; Cards edition.

CHAPTER 7—OUR CHANGING BODIES: HORMONAL AND CYCLICAL CHANGE

1. Richardson, S. F., V. Senikas, et al. 1987. "Follicular depletion during the menopausal transition: Evidence for accelerated loss and ultimate exhaustion. *J Clin Endocr Metab* 65:1231.

2. Prior, J. C. 1998. Perimenopause: The ovary's frustrating grand finale. *A Friend Indeed* 14(7):1–2.

3. Klein, N. A., P. J. Illingworth, et al. 1996. "Decreased inhibin B secretion is associated with the monotropic FSH rise in older, ovulatory women: A study of serum and follicular fluid levels of dimeric inhibin A and B in spontaneous menstrual cycles." *J Clin Endocrin Metab* 81(7):2742–45.

4. Burger, H. G., E. C. Dudley, et al. 1995. The endocrinology of the menopausal transition: A cross-sectional study of a population-based sample. *J Clin Endocrin Metab* 80:3537–45.

CHAPTER 8—MAKING INFORMED CHOICES ABOUT HORMONE REPLACEMENT THERAPY (HRT): BODY WISDOM

1. Gamble, C. 1995. Osteoporosis: Making the diagnosis in patients at risk for fracture. *Geriatrics* 50:24–33.

2. Luckey, M., D. E. Meier, et al. 1989. Radial and vertebral bone density in white and black women: evidence for racial differences in premenopausal bone homeostasis. *J Clin Endocrinol Metab* 69(4):762–70.

3. Russell-Aulet, M., et al. 1993. Bone mineral density and mass in a cross-sectional study of white and Asian women. *J Bone Miner Res* 8:575–82.

4. Warren, M. P., et al. 1986. Scoliosis and fractures in young ballet dancers: Relation to delayed menarche and secondary amenorrhea. *N Engl J Med* 314:1348–53.

5. Lloyd, T., et al. 1988. Collegiate women athletes with irregular menses during adolescence have decreased bone density. *Obstet Gynecol* 72:639–42.

6. Rigotti, N. A., R. M. Neer, et al. 1991. The clinical course of osteoporosis in anorexia nervosa: A longitudinal study of cortical bone mass. *JAMA* 265:1133–38.

7. Hudson, Tori. 1999. Women's Encyclopedia of Natural Medicine. Lincolnwood, IL: Keats, p. 196.

8. Sullivan J. M., et al. 1988. Postmenopausal estrogen use and coronary atherosclerosis. *Ann Intern Med* 108(3):358–62.

9. Herrington, D. M., et al. 1999. The HERS trial results: Paradigms lost? Heart and estrogen/progestin replacement study. *Ann Intern Med* 131(6):463–66.

10. Symeon the New Theologian (949–1022). Quoted in *The Enlightened Heart: An Anthology of Sacred Poetry.* Edited by Stephen Mitchell. New York: HarperCollins, 1989. 38–39.

11. Mark 14:23–24. Bible passage.

10. Sener, A. B., et al. 1996. The effects of hormone replacement therapy on uterine fibroids in postmenopausal women. *Fertility and Sterility* 65(2):354–57.

11. Kimzey L. M., et al. 1991. Absorption of micronized progesterone from a nonliquifying vaginal cream. *Fertility and Sterility* 56:995–96.

12. Hudson, T. 1995 (June). Estrogen replacement therapy: A guide to conventional and "quasi-natural choices. *Townsend Letter for Doctors,* pp. 164–65.

REFLECTIONS BY MARLISE WABUN WIND

1. Brooke Medicine Eagle, "Grandmother Lodge." *Wildfire* 3(4,):19–20.

CHAPTER 9—NUTRITION FOR MENOPAUSAL WOMEN: BODY ENLIGHTENMENT

1. Worthington, V. 1998. Effect of agricultural methods on nutritional quality: a comparison of organic with conventional crops. *Altern Ther Health Med* 4(1):58–69.

2. Ludwig, D. S., et al. 1999. Dietary fiber, weight gain, and cardiovascular disease risk factors in young adults. *JAMA* 282(16):1539–46.

3. Wolk, A., et al. 1999. Long-term intake of dietary fiber and decreased risk of coronary heart disease among women. *Journal of the American Medical Association* 281(21): 1998–2004.

4. Budwig, Johanna. 1992, 1994. Flax oil as a true aid against arthritis, heart infarction, cancer, and other diseases. Vancouver, BC: Apple Publishing Company, p. 7.

5. Willet, W. C., et al. 1993. Intake of *trans* fatty acids and risk of coronary heart disease among women. *Lancet* 69:3–19.

6. De Lorgeril, M., et al. 1997. Control of bias in dietary trial to prevent coronary recurrences: The Lyon diet heart study. *Eur J Clin Nutr* 51:116–22.

CHAPTER 10—EXERCISE FOR MENOPAUSAL WOMEN: MEDITATION IN MOTION

1. Hammar, M., et al. 1990. Does physical exercise influence the frequency of postmenopausal hot flushes? *Acta Obstet Gynecol Scand* 69:409–412.

2. Seals, D. R., et al. 1997. Effect of regular aerobic exercise on elevated blood pressure in postmenopausal women. *Am J Cardiol* 80:49–55.

3. Pedersen, B. K. 1991. Influence of physical activity on the cellular immune system: Mechanisms of action. *Int J Sports Med* 12, suppl. 1:S23–9.

4. Rodriguez, A. B., et al. 1991. Phagocytic function of blood neutrophils in sedentary young people after physical exercise. *Int J Sports Med* 12(3):276–80.

5. Smith, J. A., et al. 1990. Exercise, training and neutrophil microbicidal activity. *Int J Sports Med* 11(3): 179–87.

6. Van Pelt, R. E, et al. 1997. Regular exercise and the age-related decline in resting metabolic rate in women. *J Clin Endocrinol Meta* 82:3208.

7. Jakicic, J. M., et al. 1995. Prescribing exercise in multiple short bouts versus one continuous bout: Effects on adherence, cardiorespiratory fitness, and weight loss in overweight women. *Int J Obes Relat Metab Disord* 19(12): 893–901.

8. Fiatarone, M. A., et al. 1994. Exercise training and nutritional supplementation for physical frailty in very elderly people. *N Engl J Med* 330(25): 1769–75.

9. Kase, Lori Miller. 1991. Lift weight to lose it. *Vogue* 181(4):222.

10. Boorstein, Sylvia. *Don't Just Do Something, Sit There: A Mindfulness Retreat with Sylvia Boorstein.* San Francisco: Harper San Francisco, 1996. 54–56.

CHAPTER 11—AN ADDITIVE APPROACH TO BONE HEALTH: INNER AND OUTER SUPPORT STRUCTURES

1. Edwards, J., et al. 1994. Age-related osteoporosis. *Clin Ger Med* 10:575–88.

2. Sherman, H. C. 1920. Calcium requirements of maintenance in man. *J Biol Chem* 44:21–27.

3. Heaney, R. P. 1994 (June). Cofactors influencing the calcium requirement—Other nutrients. Paper presented at the NIH Consensus Development Conference on Optimal Calcium Intake, Bethesda, MD, June 1994.

4. Breslau, N. A., et al. 1988. Relationship of animal protein-rich diet, kidney stone formation and calcium metabolism. *J Clin Endocrinol Metabol* 66:140–46.

5. Hernandez-Avila, M., et al. 1991. Caffeine, moderate alcohol intake, and risk of fractures of the hip and forearm in middle-aged women. *Am J Clin Nutr* 54:157–63.

6. Wyshak, G., and R. E. Frisch. 1994. Carbonated beverages, dietary calcium, the dietary calcium/phosphorus ration, and bone fractures in girls and boys. *Adolesc Health* 15(3):210–15.

7. Mazariegos-Ramos, E., et al. 1995. Consumption of soft drinks with phosphoric acid as a risk factor for hypocalcemia in children: A case-control study. *J Pediatr* 126:940–42.

8. Rockwell, J., et al. 1990. Weight training decreases vertebral bone density in premenopausal women: A prospective study. *J Clin Endocrinol Metab* 71:988.

9. Jaglal, S., et al. 1993. Post and recent physical activity and risk of hip fractures. *Am J Epid* 138:107.

10. Henderson, N. K., C. P. White, and J. A. Eisman. 1998. The roles of exercise and fall risk reduction in the prevention of osteoporosis. *Endocrinol Metab Clin North Am*

27(2): 369–87.

11. Lane, N., et al. 1996. Long-distance running, bone density, and osteoarthritis. *JAMA* 255:1147.

12. Stillman, R. J., et al. 1986. Physical activity and bone mineral content in women aged 30 to 85 years. *Med Sci Sports Exerc* 18(5):576–80.

13. Heaney, R. 1996. Bone mass, nutrition, and other lifestyle factors. *Nutr Rev* 54:53.

14. Bassey, E. 1995. Exercise in primary prevention of osteoporosis in women. *Ann Rheum Dis* 54:861.

15. Chow, R., et al. 1987. Effect of two randomised exercise programmes on bone mass in healthy postmenopausal women. *Br Med J* 295:1441.

16. Pruitt, L., et al. 1995. Effects of a one-year high-intensity versus low-intensity resistance training program on bone mineral density in older women. *J Bone Miner Res* 10:1788.

17. American College of Sports Medicine. 1995. ACSM position stand on osteoporosis and exercise. *Med Sci Sports Exerc* 27:i–vii.

18. Bloomfield, S. A., et al. 1993. Non-weightbearing exercise may increase lumbar spine bone mineral density in healthy postmenopausal women. *Am J Phys Med Rehabil* 72(4):204–9.

19. DeBenedette, V. 1987. Swimming may increase bone density. *The Physician and Sportsmedicine* 15(12):49.

20. Kohrt, W. M., A. A. Ehsani, and S. J. Birge, Jr. 1997. Effects of exercise involving predominantly either joint-reaction or ground-reaction forces on bone mineral density in older women. *J Bone Miner Res* 12(8):1253–61.

21. Brewer, V., B. M. Meyer, M. S. Keele, S. J. Upton, and R. D. Hagan. 1983. Role of exercise in prevention of involutional bone loss. *Med Sci Sports Exerc* 15(6):445–49.

22. Sinaki, M., and K. P. Offord. 1988. Physical activity in postmenopausal women: Effect on back muscle strength and bone mineral density of the spine. *Arch Phys Med Rehabil* 69(4): 277–80.

23. Fiatarone, M.A. et al. 1994. Exercise training and nutritional supplementation for physical frailty in very elderly people. *N Engl J Med* 330(25):1769–75.

24. Flatz, G. 1987. Genetics of lactose digestion in humans. In *Harris, H., and K. Hirschorn (eds.), Advances in Human Genetics*. New York: Plenum, pp. 1–77.

25. Weaver, C. M., and K. L. Plawecki. 1994. Dietary calcium: Adequacy of a vegetarian diet. *Am J Clin Nutr* 59(suppl):12385–415.

26. Grossman, M., et al. 1963. Basal and histalog-stimulated gasric secretion in control subjects and in patients with peptic ulcer or gastric cancer. *Gastroent* 45:15–26.

27. Cumming, R. G., S. R. Cummings, M.C. Nevitt, et al. 1997. Calcium intake and fracture risk: Results from the study of osteoporotic fractures. *Am J Epidemiol* 145:926–34.

28. Feskanich, D., W. C. Willett, et al. Milk, dietary calcium, and bone fractures in women: A 12-year prospective study. *Am J Public Health* 87:992–97.

29. Nielsen, F. 1988. Boron—An overlooked element of potential nutritional importance. *Nutr Today* January/February:4–7.

30. Wilcox, Ella Wheeler. The Winds of Faith. *Poems of Optimism.* Whitefish, MT: Kessinger Publishing: 2004. 16.

CHAPTER 12—RITUALS TO MARK THE MENOPAUSAL JOURNEY: RITES AND CELEBRATIONS

1. Price, Len and Shirley. 1999. *Aromatherapy for Health Professionals, Second Ed..* New York: Churchill Livingston. 210–15.

2. Walker, B. G. 1985. *The Crone.* San Francisco: Harper & Row.

3. Cameron, A. 1981. *Daughters of Copper Woman.* Vancouver, B. C.: Press Gang Publishers.

4. "Centering Home" and "All One Planet." 1991. Recorded on the Sumitra Music label, Box 327, Charlemont, MA 01339. Discography available at www.mollyscot.com.

5. Emoto, M., and D. A. Thayne. 2004. *Messages from Water.* Gallatin, TN: Source Books.

6. "All One Planet." 1991. Lyrics by Molly Scott. Recorded on the Sumitra Music label, Box 327, Charlemont, MA 01339. Discography available at www.mollyscot.com.

BIBLIOGRAPHY

Boice, Judith. The Pocket Guide to Naturopathic Medicine. Berkeley: Crossing Press, 1996.

Boice, Judith: "But My Doctor Never Told Me That!": secrets for creating lifelong health. Portland, OR: Althea Press, 1999.

Boice, Judith, editor. Mother Earth: Through the Eyes of Women Photographers and Writers. San Francisco: Sierra Club Books, 2002.

Bridges, Carol. The Code of the Goddess, Sacred Earth: feng shui oracle. Indiana: Earth Nations Publishing, 2001

Bridges, Carol. Medicine Woman Tarot (card deck). Connecticut: U.S. Game Systems, Inc., 1989.

Cameron, Anne. Daughters of Copper Woman. Madeira Park, B.C.: Harbour Publishing Ltd., 1981.

Estès, Clarissa Pinkola. Women Who Run With The Wolves. New York: Ballantine, 1996.

Estès, Clarissa Pinkola. The Faithful Gardener: a wise tale about that which can never die. San Francisco: HarperSanFrancisco, 1995.

Flinders, Carol. Enduring Lives: portraits of women and faith in action. New York: Tarcher, 2006.

Flinders, Carol. At the Root of This Longing: reconciling a spiritual hunger and a feminist thirst. San Francisco: HarperSanFrancisco, 1998.

Medicine Eagle, Brooke. Buffalo Woman Comes Singing. New York: Ballantine, 1991.

Medicine Eagle, Brooke. The Last Ghost Dance: a guide for earth mages. New York: Ballantine, 2000.

Noble, Vicki. Motherpeace:A Way to the Goddess Through Myth, Art, and Tarot. New York: HarperCollins, 1983.

Noble, Vicki. Shakti Woman: feeling our fire, healing our world – the new female shamanism. New York: HarperCollins, 1991.

Noble, Vicki. The Double Goddess: women sharing power. Vermont: Bear & Company, 2003.

Walker, Barbara. Crone: woman of age, wisdom, and power. San Francisco: HarperSanFrancisco, 1988.

Wind, Marlise Wabun. Woman of the Dawn. New York: Prentice Hall. 1989.

Wind, Marlise Wabun. The Medicine Wheel: earth astrology. New York: Fireside. 1980.

INDEX